PERIODONTAL EXAMINATION

JAN EGELBERG

ANITA BADERSTEN

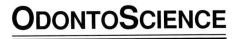
ODONTO**S**CIENCE

Periodontal Examination
1st edition, 2nd printing

Copyright © 1997 Odonto Science, Malmö, Sweden

Drawings by Pia Lindgren

Cover composition by Tegnestuen

Text editing by Noel Claffey

Printed in Sweden by Team Offset & Media, Malmö

ISBN: 91-971823-2-X

The authors acknowledge the following for contribution of illustrations:
Anna-Lisa Björn (Fig. 43, 44, 48, 54)
Bernard Gantes (Fig. 63, 64, 66, 70, 71)
Björn Klinge (Fig. 10, 26)
Lars Matsson (Fig. 6, 24)
Stefan Renvert (Fig. 57, 61, 62)
Bengt Sjödin (Fig. 76)
Björn Svensson (Fig. 12)
Göran Söderholm (Fig. 46)
Gunilla Tynelius-Bratthall (Fig. 50)
Anna Örnhall-Britse (Fig. 36)

Contents

Preface

This textbook describes:

- the structures of the periodontal tissues;

- the alterations occurring in gingivitis and periodontitis; and

- current methods for periodontal examination.

The book is written for students of dentistry of any category. The basic elements of the periodontal examination are described with the aid of pertinent illustrations. Questions for self-assessment have been added to each section. A list of terms and their explanations is included at the end of the book to help those who are unfamiliar with periodontal terms.

We hope that the reader will find the book both instructive and easy to understand.

Jan Egelberg   *Anita Badersten*

The healthy periodontium

The supporting structures of the tooth are collectively termed the periodontium and include:

gingiva
periodontal ligament
cementum
alveolar bone (Fig. 1).

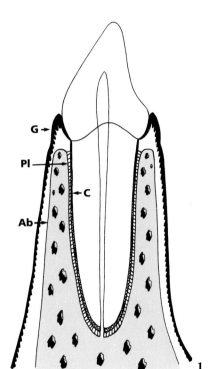

Fig. 1. Schematic illustration of the periodontium. G=gingiva, Pl=periodontal ligament, Ab=alveolar bone, C=cementum.

Gingival anatomy

The gingiva covers the alveolar bone and surrounds the teeth. The gingival margin forms the coronal extension of the gingiva on the buccal and lingual aspects of the teeth. The margin follows a wavy course across the dentition due to the interdental papillae, which fill the interdental spaces beneath the tooth contacts (Fig. 2, p. 8; Fig. 15, p. 17).

Fig. 2. Healthy gingiva in the mandibular anterior region.

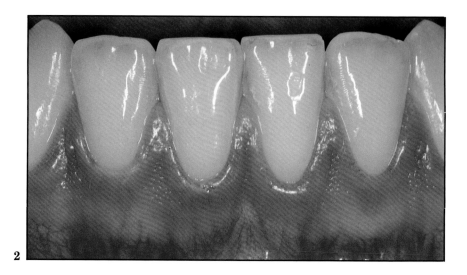

2

Interdental papilla

The shape of the interdental papilla is determined by the tooth contacts, the widths of the neighboring teeth, and the curvature of the cementoenamel junction. The buccolingual dimensions of the papillae are narrower in the anterior than in the posterior areas. Accordingly, the papillae are more pyramid-shaped anteriorly and wider buccolingually for posterior areas (Fig. 3a, 3b).

The coronal extension of the interdental papilla often consists of buccal and lingual peaks with a col between the two peaks. In this way the papilla embraces the contacts of adjacent teeth (Fig. 3a, 3b).

Fig. 3a, 3b. Illustration of the difference in shape of the interdental papilla in anterior and posterior areas.

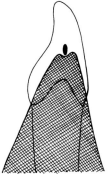 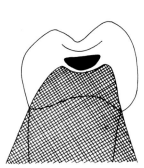

3a, 3b

Apically, the gingiva extends to the mucogingival junction: the demarcation between the gingiva and the alveolar mucosa (Fig. 2, p. 8; Fig. 4a-4c).

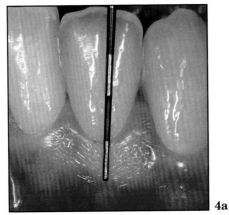

4a

The width (height) of the gingiva varies in the dentition between 1-9 mm. The buccal gingiva in the maxilla is usually widest in the anterior region and narrowest in the premolar area. On the palatal aspect, the maxillary gingiva merges with the palatal mucosa without a demarcation line. In the mandible, the buccal gingiva is generally widest in the incisor region and narrowest in the cuspid and premolar areas. On the lingual aspect, the mandibular gingiva is widest in the premolar and molar regions and narrowest in the anterior areas.

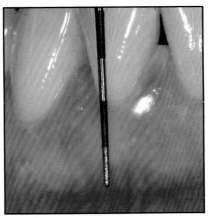

4b

Two portions of the gingiva can be identified:

- free marginal gingiva
- attached gingiva.

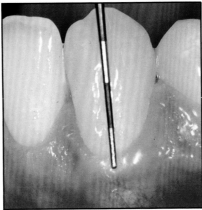

4c

Mucogingival junction

Fig. 4a-4c. Examples showing variation of the gingival width between different individuals and between different regions of the dentition.

Gingival width

Free marginal gingiva

The free marginal gingiva includes the interdental papillae and and the coronal gingiva to a level approximating the cemento-enamel junction. In some individuals, the apical extension is demarcated with a furrow: the gingival groove (Fig. 5).

Attached gingiva

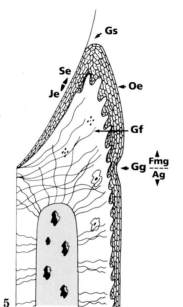

Fig. 5. Illustration of the free marginal gingiva (Fmg) and the attached gingiva (Ag). Gs=gingival sulcus, Oe=oral epithelium, Se=sulcular epithelium, Je=junctional epithelium, Gg=gingival groove, Gf=gingival fibers.

The attached gingiva extends from the level of the gingival groove apically to the mucogingival junction, where the gingiva merges with the alveolar mucosa. The attached gingiva is firmly bound to the underlying cementum and bone with collagen fibers of the connective tissue.

Alveolar mucosa

The alveolar mucosa is loosely attached to the underlying bone and has a brighter red color (Fig. 2, p. 8; Fig. 26, p. 38).

Gingival epithelium

The gingival epithelium can be divided into:
- oral epithelium
- sulcular epithelium
- junctional epithelium (or dentogingival epithelium).

The oral epithelium extends from the gingival margin to the mucogingival junction. The sulcular epithelium faces the tooth. Apical to the sulcular epithelium, the gingiva is joined to the tooth by the junctional epithelium.

Gingival sulcus

A sulcus - the gingival sulcus - is formed at the gingival margin and bordered by the sulcular epithelium and the tooth surface.

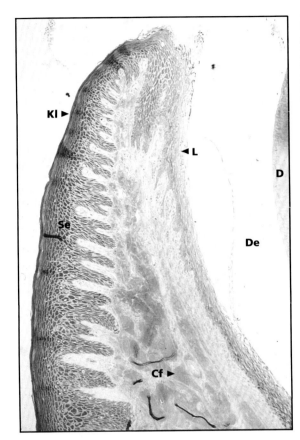
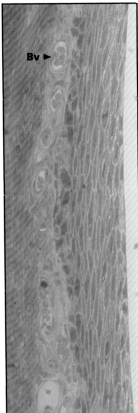

Fig. 6a, 6b. Histological preparations of clinically healthy gingiva. Slight epithelial proliferation and cellular infiltration can be seen in the sulcular region. Fig. 6b is a magnification of the apical part of the dentogingival epithelium in Fig. 6a. Stratified, keratinized squamous epithelium (Se), keratin layer (Kl), collagen fiber bundles (Cf), leukocytes (L), demineralized enamel (De), dentin (D), blood vessels (Bv).

6a, 6b

Oral epithelium

The oral epithelium is stratified and includes several layers of cells. The basal cells are columnar in shape, the middle cells more hexagonal and the superficial cells flattened and keratinized (stratified, keratinized squamous epithelium). Epithelial ridges and mounds interface with connective tissue projections.

Sulcular epithelium

The sulcular epithelium is similar to the oral epithelium, but loses the keratinized layer as the cells contact the tooth surface.

Junctional epithelium

The junctional epithelium is comparatively thin and has an even interface with the connective tissue. In the apical part it may include only a few layers of cells, whereas in the coronal part it may include 15-30 layers. The cells are somewhat flattened, do not keratinize and have wide intercellular spaces. Bacterial products can pass into the connective tissue through this permeable epithelium, and antibody-containing tissue fluids can ooze out. Inflammatory cells can migrate through the epithelium. Polymorphonuclear leukocytes can often be seen between the epithelial cells, migrating towards the sulcular region - also under healthy conditions (Fig. 6a, 6b, p. 11).

Mucosal epithelium

The epithelium of the alveolar mucosa is often thinner than the oral epithelium and lacks keratinization. The projections (rete pegs) into the connective tissue are generally smaller and may also be absent. The translucent nonkeratinized epithelium allows the underlying blood vessels to be seen, explaining the brighter red color of the mucosa (Fig. 2, p. 8; Fig. 4a-4c, p. 9).

Collagen fibers

Fig. 7. Illustration of the groups of collagen fibers of the gingiva.

Dentogingival fibers (Dg): originate from the supra-alveolar cementum around the tooth and spread coronally into the gingiva.

Alveologingival fibers (Ag): spread from the alveolar bone into the gingiva.

Alveolodental fibers (Ad): the fibers of the periodontal ligament connecting the cementum and the alveolar bone.

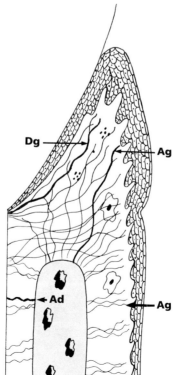

Gingival connective tissue

The connective tissue of the gingiva consists of dense networks of collagen fibers. These provide the tonus (firmness) of the gingiva and the attachment to the cementum and alveolar bone. The fibers project in different directions to ensure an adequate gingival anchorage (Fig. 7; Fig. 8a, 8b, p. 13).

Apart from fibers, the connective tissue consists of blood and lymphatic vessels, nerves, cells and ground substance. The main cell - the fibroblast - produces both collagen fibers and ground substance. In the connective tissue next to the sulcular region, some inflammatory cells can be found (polymorphonuclear leukocytes, monocytes, lymphocytes and plasma cells).

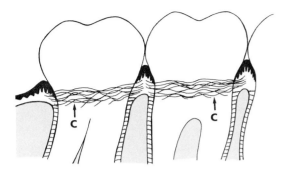

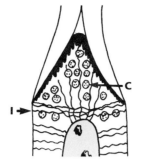

8a, 8b

Fig. 8a. Circular fibers (C): extend around the tooth in the free marginal gingiva, intertwine and provide a cuff-like arrangement.

Fig. 8b. Interdental (I) or transseptal fibers: extend from the supra-alveolar cementum of one tooth, pass through the interdental gingiva and attach to the cementum of the adjacent tooth.

Gingival crevice

A gingival crevice may be created, extending apically from the gingival margin. Normally, the junctional epithelium adheres to the tooth and no crevice is present. A crevice becomes apparent if an instrument, such as a periodontal probe, penetrates apically along the tooth surface (Fig. 9).

For a normal periodontium, the periodontal probe will stop at the cemento-enamel junction or slightly coronally. The extent of probe penetration depends on the diameter of the probe tip, the probing force and the tonus of the gingival connective tissue. After successful treatment of periodontitis, a healthy gingival crevice may be located more apically on the root surface.

The normal probing depth (crevicular depth) is usually 1-3 mm. Approximal sites generally have the deepest normal probing depths, followed by the lingual sites. Buccal sites usually have the shallowest probing depths.

Fig. 9. Probing normal gingiva. The probe tip displaces the junctional epithelium. The probing depth (crevicular depth) illustrated amounts to 2.5 mm.

9

Periodontal ligament

Periodontal ligament

The periodontal ligament embraces the entire root to a level 1-1.5 mm apical to the cementoenamel junction. The ligament is generally 0.2-0.5 mm wide and contains bundles of collagen fibers anchoring the tooth to the alveolar bone. The fibers extend from the cementum to the bone and are embedded into these calcified tissues at both ends. A wavy arrangement of the fibers permit a slight, normal mobility for the tooth (Fig. 10).

Cementum

The dentin of the root is covered by a layer of cementum. The thickness of the cementum varies. Close to the cementoenamel junction it may amount to only 0.1 mm in thickness. Apically, it may approach 1 mm.

Acellular and cellular cementum

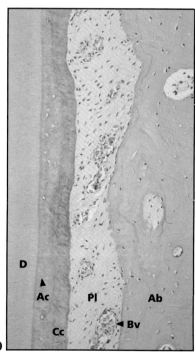

Fig. 10. Histological section of a periodontal ligament. Dentin (D), cellular cementum (Cc) with several empty lacunae due to cell death, acellular cementum (Ac), periodontal ligament (Pl), blood vessels (Bv), alveolar bone (Ab).

Two types of cementum can be distinguished: acellular and cellular (without and with cells). The acellular cementum is found next to the dentin and is formed during the development of the tooth. Cellular cementum, which includes cementocytes in lacunae, is deposited on top of the acellular cementum during function (Fig. 10). The cementum serves to anchor the periodontal ligament fibers to the tooth.

Alveolar process

The alveolar process provides the housing for the dental roots. The coronal margin of the alveolar bone extends across the dentition with a wavy configuration, corresponding to the course of the cementoenamel junctions of the teeth, and at a distance of 1-1.5 mm from these junctions (Fig. 11a, 11b).

The alveolar process consists of a buccal and a lingual plate of compact bone. The sockets for the teeth (alveolae) are also lined with compact bone that is visible in dental radiographs and termed lamina dura. This layer anchors the periodontal ligament fibers. Blood vessels and nerves penetrate through the layer and supply the ligament. The interior of the alveolar process contains cancellous bone with bony trabeculae and bone marrow (Fig. 12).

Lamina dura

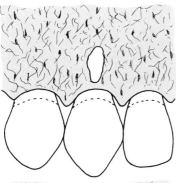

The thickness of the alveolar process varies throughout the dentition and is partly a function of the buccolingual width of the teeth. At times, there may be a lack of bony coverage of the roots, primarily in teeth positioned buccally or lingually in the dental arch (Fig. 11a, 11b).

Fig. 11a, 11b. Illustration of the wavy course of the alveolar margin and examples of lack of bony root coverage. 11a: fenestration; 11b: dehiscence.

11a

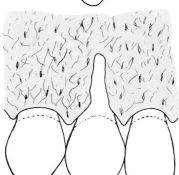

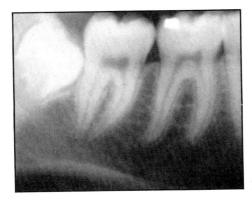

Fig 12. Radiographic image of the alveolar process in the mandibular posterior region (with an unerupted third molar). Compact and cancellous bone can be identified.

11b, 12

Periodontal blood vessels

Fig. 13 presents a schematic illustration of the blood supply to the teeth and the periodontal tissues. Larger vessels gradually branch into vascular networks with numerous interconnections (anastomoses) nourishing the various parts of the periodontium.

Capillary loops
Dentogingival plexus

The peripheral gingival blood supply underlying the oral and sulcular epithelia is composed of capillary loops located within the connective tissue projections. Next to the junctional epithelium there is a network of peripheral blood vessels termed the dentogingival plexus (Fig. 14).

Fig. 13. Schematic illustration of the periodontal blood vessels. Main vessels to the alveolar process (A), vascular network of the periodontal ligament (P), dentogingival plexus (Dgp), compact bone (Cb).

Fig. 14. Histological preparation demonstrating the gingival blood vessels underneath the oral (Oe) and sulcular epithelia and adjacent to the unstained junctional epithelium (Je). Capillary loops (Cl), dentogingival plexus (Dgp).

13, 14

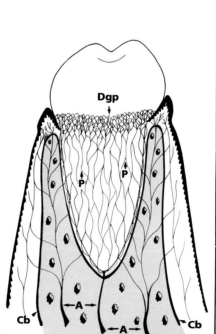

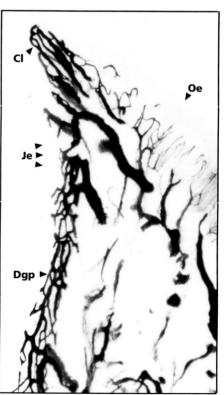

Clinical signs of healthy gingiva

The healthy gingiva (Fig. 15) is pink or light red in color. Individual color variations exist, related to the thickness of the epithelium and the presence of pigmented cells (melanocytes). Pigmented gingiva is often seen in individuals with a dark complexion.

Color

The gingival surface may show small depressions giving it a stippled appearance like an orange peel. Approximately 40% of individuals with healthy gingiva have been found to exhibit a stippled gingival surface.

Surface texture

The gingival margin is thin and follows a wavy course across the dentition due to the presence of the interdental papillae, which fill the embrasures between the teeth. The overall gingival form is governed by the shape of the teeth, the tooth contacts, the width of the alveolar bone and the course of the coronal bone margin.

Contour

The tonus of the free gingiva is firm due to the presence of dense networks of collagen fibers.

Tonus

The probing depth is usually ≤3 mm (Fig. 9, p. 13).

Probing depth

Following probing of the gingival crevice with a gentle force, bleeding is usually absent or limited.

Bleeding on probing

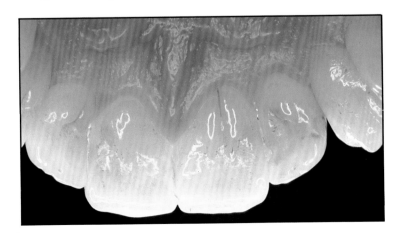

Fig. 15. Healthy gingiva on the palatal aspect of maxillary anterior teeth.

15

The healthy periodontium

Questions

1. Which tissue components form the periodontium?

2. Describe the following structures:
   a) gingiva
   b) gingival margin
   c) interdental papilla
   d) mucogingival junction.

3. Describe some variations of gingival width in the dentition.

4. What features characterize
   a) the free marginal gingiva?
   b) the attached gingiva?
   c) the alveolar mucosa?

5. List the different types of gingival epithelia.

6. Describe the gingival sulcus.

7. Describe the histological structure of
   a) the oral epithelium
   b) the sulcular epithelium
   c) the junctional epithelium
   d) the epithelium of the alveolar mucosa.

8. Describe the various groups of collagen fibers present in the gingiva.

9. Define the terms gingival crevice and crevicular depth.

10. What is the probing depth of the normal gingival crevice and how does it vary around the tooth?

11. Describe the periodontal ligament.

12. What are the characteristics of the different types of cementum?

13. Which are the bony components of the alveolar process and what are their characteristics?

14. Describe the blood supply to the periodontal tissues.

15. What is the dentogingival plexus?

16. List the clinical signs used to evaluate gingival health.

17. Describe the characteristics of healthy gingiva in terms of
    a) color
    b) surface texture
    c) contour
    d) tonus
    e) probing depth
    f) bleeding on probing.

Dental plaque and calculus

Supragingival plaque

Following a few days without toothbrushing, dental plaque forms on the teeth to the extent that it can be observed with the naked eye.

Dental plaque usually first forms at the gingival margin, particularly on the approximal surfaces. In these areas the plaque build-up is protected by the contours of the teeth and the gingiva. Without toothbrushing, the plaque gradually increases in thickness and spreads coronally over the crown.

Initial plaque formation

The rate of plaque formation varies from one individual to another. Usually, plaque forms more quickly in the posterior than in the anterior areas. A rough tooth surface favors plaque growth rather than a smooth surface (Fig. 16a, 16b, p. 20).

Rate of plaque formation

The coronal growth and extension of the plaque is related to the amount of wear from the lips, the cheek and the tongue. A hard or fibrous diet may have little effect on the growth of plaque along the gingival margin and interdentally but may have some effect on coronal tooth surfaces.

Coronal plaque extension

Supragingival calculus

Calcium salts may be deposited in the supragingival plaque, resulting in mineralization of the plaque and formation of calculus. Supragingival calculus is primarily formed on the lingual surfaces of the mandibular anterior teeth but sometimes also on the buccal surfaces of the maxillary molars. Saliva from the major salivary ducts enters the oral cavity in these areas and creates a biochemical environment favoring mineral deposition. For this reason, supragingival calculus is also termed salivary calculus. In some individuals, salivary calculus may be formed and visible as soon as a week or two after the teeth have been cleaned (Fig. 17, p. 21).

Salivary calculus

Initially, supragingival calculus is white-yellow, somewhat grainy and brittle. Litte by little, it becomes darker due to discoloration and harder due to increased mineralization.

Fig. 16a, 16b. Dental plaque shown by use of a plaque-disclosing dye in a person who has refrained from toothbrushing.
16a: after 2 days; 16b: after 4 days.

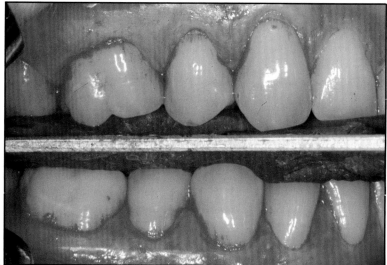

16a

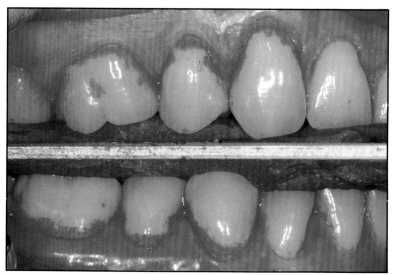

16b

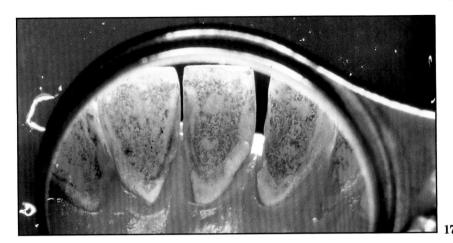

Fig. 17. Supragingival calculus at the gingival margin on the lingual aspects of mandibular incisors. More coronally, thin, stained, noncalculus deposits are seen.

Subgingival plaque

From its initial location at the gingival margin, the plaque gradually extends apically. Plaque located adjacent to the gingiva causes inflammation of the gingival tissues. This results in decreased adaptation of the marginal gingiva to the tooth, which facilitates initial subgingival colonization. The continued apical penetration of the microorganisms occurs along pathways offering least resistance. Gradually, the plaque coalesces into subgingival bacterial masses.

Apical extension of plaque

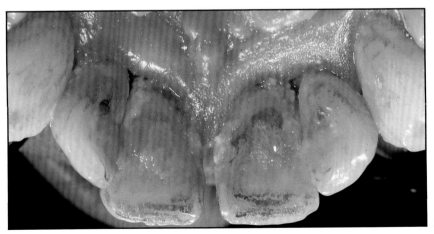

18

Fig. 18. Abundance of supragingival plaque on the palatal surfaces of the maxillary incisors. Dark areas can be seen underneath the plaque adjacent to the gingival margin, where calculus, previously located subgingivally, has become visible following gingival recession.

Gradual subgingival penetration

Subgingival growth and penetration of plaque is a slow process. It is the result of neglected plaque control along the gingival margin over extended periods of time. In individuals with initially healthy gingiva, it probably takes several months of undisturbed plaque at the gingival margin before the plaque has established itself subgingivally to the extent that it no longer can be removed with the toothbrush. At this stage, removal requires professional intervention. If plaque is allowed to re-accumulate at the gingival margin after recent debridement of inflamed periodontal pockets, subgingival re-colonization will take place within a shorter time, perhaps within 1-2 months.

Development of gingivitis and periodontitis

The supragingival plaque causes inflammation of the marginal periodontal tissues: gingivitis. Apical penetration of the plaque causes inflammation of the deeper periodontal tissues: periodontitis.

Subgingival calculus

Subgingival mineralization

Serumal calculus

Mineralization of subgingival plaque can take place at any location in the dentition where there has been sufficient subgingival growth. The minerals required for calcification originate in the inflammatory exudate (of serumal origin), which oozes into periodontal pockets from inflamed gingival tissues. For this reason, subgingival calculus is also termed serumal calculus.

Subgingival calculus may be detected by probing the tooth surface within periodontal pockets and by radiographic examination. Subgingival mineralization is a slow process. Several years of continuous presence of subgingival plaque may be required before mineralization has progressed sufficiently to allow the calculus to be detected.

Subgingival calculus is most often seen on approximal surfaces. These surfaces are more difficult to clean and are often continuously overlooked during toothbrushing, thus favoring the subgingival colonization of bacteria. Subgingival calculus is usually dark and hard when it is discovered. Mineralization first occurs at multiple sites in small amounts, which makes detection of the calculus at the early stages difficult.

In plaque-infected subgingival areas that have remained undisturbed for years, only about one third of the total plaque area is mineralized. Following gingival recession, subgingival calculus may become exposed and visible (Fig. 18, p. 21; Fig. 39a, 40a, 40b, p. 53). Occasionally, patients who do not seem to form subgingival calculus can be encountered.

Adequate treatment requires complete removal of both mineralized and nonmineralized supra- and subgingival plaque. In patients with periodontitis, calculus has formed on the naturally uneven root surfaces, and debridement may be both difficult and time-consuming. In patients with gingivitis, debridement is comparatively easy, as calculus is present primarily on the smoother enamel surfaces.

Recording supragingival plaque

Records of supragingival plaque are obtained to reflect the ability of individual patients to perform plaque control. A series of consecutive recordings performed at intervals following oral hygiene instruction is useful for evaluation of the effectiveness of the routines recommended.

Dental plaque has a white-yellow color, similar to the teeth. Red plaque-disclosing dyes can be used to facilitate detection. Only deeply stained areas should be recorded. Films of precipitated salivary proteins (pellicle) will also stain slightly and should not be included.

Disclosing dyes

Salivary pellicle

If disclosing dyes are not used, the teeth should be dried with compressed air to allow the detection of plaque. The tip of a probe, moved along the tooth surface, will facilitate plaque recognition.

Probe tip

Different recording systems are used. Some of these reflect the presence or absence of plaque at the gingival margin. Other methods score the amounts and/or the extension of the plaque on the tooth surfaces. The Plaque Index according to Silness & Löe considers plaque at the gingival margin only and grades the amounts of plaque in these locations as follows:

0 = no plaque;

1 = small amounts of plaque visible after use of disclosing dye or by running a probe tip along the gingival margin;

2 = moderate amounts of plaque that can be seen with the naked eye;

3 = abundance of plaque.

Plaque Index

The Plaque Index for the individual patient is calculated by adding the scores for each examined tooth surface and dividing by the number of examined surfaces.

A plaque score based on the presence or absence of plaque at the gingival margin may be most common in clinical practice. The presence of plaque is recorded for 4 or 6 surfaces of each tooth. A percentage score is calculated for the patient by dividing the number of surfaces with plaque by the total number of examined surfaces.

Recording subgingival plaque and calculus

Detection of subgingival plaque and calculus is often difficult. Routine recordings systems are not applicable. The subgingival examination may therefore be limited to a number of attempts at finding plaque or calculus in different locations of the dentition.

Examination for subgingival plaque

Examination for *nonmineralized subgingival plaque* can be performed as follows:

• Dry the area with compressed air and observe the gingiva. An inflamed gingiva that bleeds easily on probing is a sign of subgingival infection.

• Remove the supragingival plaque with a suitable instrument or with a cotton pellet. Probe the subgingival area and try to retrieve any plaque with the probe tip.

Examination for *subgingival calculus* can be performed as follows:

• Look for any calculus present in the orifice of the periodontal pockets. The marginal gingiva may appear blue if the gingiva is thin enough to allow reflection of the dark serumal calculus.

• Insert the probe into the pocket and widen the orifice by angling the probe away from the tooth. This may allow inspection. A carefully directed jet of compressed air may also open up the pocket somewhat for inspection.

• Probe the subgingival area, up and down, with zig-zag movements. Try to find rough areas.

Subgingival calculus on approximal surfaces of the teeth may show on radiographs. With X-ray projection suitable for approximal surfaces, the calculus may be recognized as small radiopaque spurs of varying shapes. Small amounts of calculus will not give enough contrast for visibility, particularly if the X-ray projection is less than optimal (Fig. 19-21; Fig. 76a-76d, p. 78).

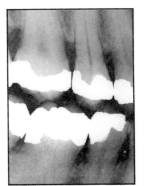 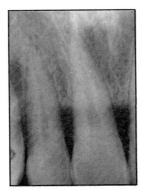 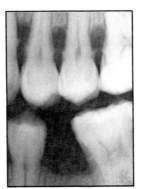

Fig. 19-21. Calculus on approximal surfaces close to the cementoenamel junction.

19, 20, 21

Dental plaque and calculus

Questions

1. On which parts of a recently cleaned tooth will dental plaque start to form? Why?

2. What variations in the rate of plaque formation and surface spread can be observed in different regions of the dentition?

3. What is supragingival calculus?

4. What is salivary calculus?

5. How is salivary calculus formed?

6. In what parts of the dentition can salivary calculus be found?

7. Describe the properties of salivary calculus.

8. Describe the development of subgingival plaque.

9. How is subgingival calculus formed?

10. What is another term for subgingival calculus?

11. In what parts of the dentition can subgingival calculus be found?

12. Describe the properties of subgingival calculus.

13. How can the detection of supragingival plaque be facilitated?

14. Describe different systems for recording supragingival plaque.

15. Describe how subgingival plaque can be detected.

16. Describe how subgingival calculus can be detected.

17. Describe the radiographic appearance of subgingival calculus.

18. Which conditions limit the possibility of radiographic detection of subgingival calculus?

Gingivitis

Inflammation of the gingiva - gingivitis - is caused by accumulation of dental plaque on the teeth. In the absence of adequate tooth-cleaning, plaque is formed at the gingival margin and on approximal surfaces. In these locations, the contours of the teeth and gingiva facilitate the retention of salivary microorganisms. Gradually, the plaque increases in thickness and extends over the tooth surfaces. Plaque left undisturbed at the gingival margin will cause an inflammatory reaction of the gingiva already within 3-4 days. The degree of inflammation will increase, and after 1-2 weeks, gingivitis can be observed at clinical examination (Fig. 22a, 22b, p. 28).

Gingivitis is caused by plaque

Gingivitis is reversible, that is, it may disappear and the gingiva may become healthy again, provided the teeth are cleaned and subsequently kept free from plaque. Most cases of gingivitis will heal within 1-2 months. Untreated gingivitis and continuous penetration of the plaque subgingivally may lead to injury to the supporting structures of the teeth (periodontal ligament, cementum and alveolar bone). Periodontitis may develop.

Gingivitis is reversible

In gingivitis, changes take place both in the epithelium and in the connective tissue (Fig. 23a-23d, pp. 30-31). Inflammatory cells accumulate in the connective tissue, initially adjacent to the gingival sulcus. Polymorphonuclear leukocytes are found close to the epithelium. Lymphocytes and plasma cells predominate in the deeper layers of the connective tissue. The polymorphonuclear leukocytes migrate towards the microbial deposits. As they migrate, they may engulf isolated bacteria that have pen-etrated into the epithelium or into the connective tissue (phagocytosis). Lymphocytes and plasma cells are activated by microbial products (antigens) and result in the production of antibodies and other immune components. Monocytes, capable of developing into macrophages, also participate in the inflammatory reaction.

Periodontitis

Accumulation of inflammatory cells

**Collagen breakdown
Vascular changes**

The collagen fibers in the connective tissue gradually disintegrate. Tissue fluids accumulate in the connective tissue (edema). The gingiva becomes clinically edematous (swollen) and the stippling on the surface may disappear. There is an increase in the number of patent blood vessels and their diameters widen. The permeability of the vessels also increases, allowing more serum and inflammatory cells (exudate) to pass through the vascular walls and accumulate in the tissue.

Inflammatory exudate

**Proliferation and
degeneration of
sulcular and
junctional epithelia**

The sulcular epthelium and the coronal part of the junctional epithelium show both proliferative and degenerative changes. Epithelial rete pegs are formed and penetrate into the connective tissue. Thinning of the epithelium takes place, sometimes to the extent that ulceration may develop and expose the connective tissue directly to the subgingival microbial deposits.

Fig. 22a, 22b. Gingivitis. Plaque along the gingival margins and interdentally; redness and some swelling of the marginal gingiva and the papillae; localized bleeding between right lateral incisor and cuspid (22a). Gentle probing of the gingival sulci of the incisors resulted in bleeding and dispersion of blood along the gingival margins (22b).

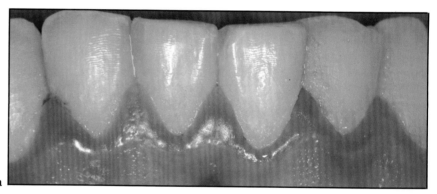

22a

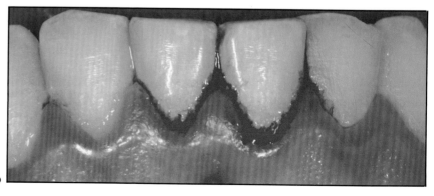

22b

Within the epithelium bordering the subgingival plaque, inflammatory cells, particularly polymorphonuclear leukocytes, are seen. The migration of these cells is facilitated by the widening of the junctions between the epithelial cells induced by the inflammatory reaction.

The plaque continues to penetrate subgingivally, and the inflammation gradually extends apically. The depth of the tissue changes is related to the degree of apical plaque penetration (Fig. 23a-23d, pp. 30-31; Fig. 24, p. 32).

Vascular changes

The vascular changes in gingivitis include altered vascular topography, increased vascular permeability and increased vascular fragility.

The course of the blood vessels changes and the number of vessels increases: vascular proliferation. The diameter of the vessels also increases. The network of vessels in gingival health, forming the dentogingival plexus, is transformed into a system with abundant vascular loops (Fig. 23a-23d, pp. 30-31; Fig. 25, p. 33).

Altered vascular topography

The increase of vascular permeability leads to accumulation of fluids and inflammatory cells in the tissues and to exudation of fluids and cells into the gingival sulcus.

Increased vascular permeability

Vascular walls rupture more easily, resulting in easily elicited bleeding. Bleeding on toothbrushing is a useful warning signal, informing the patient that inflammation may be present. In cases of more severe gingivitis, spontaneous bleeding may also occur. The tendency to bleed in gingivitis is explained by increased fragility of vessels located more superficially beneath thinned areas of the sulcular and junctional epithelia.

Increased vascular fragility

*Fig. 23a-23d. For legends,
see p. 31.*

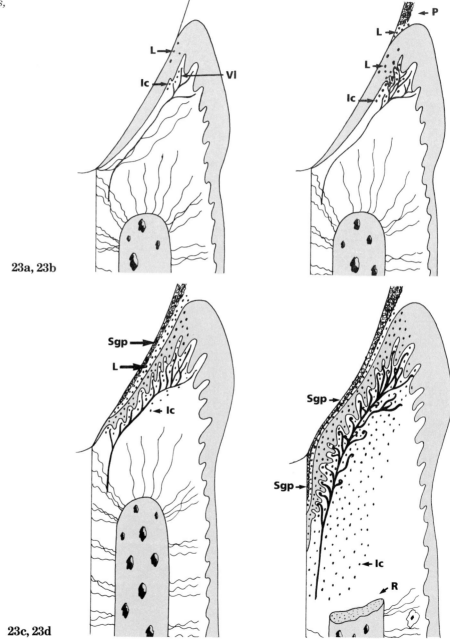

23a, 23b

23c, 23d

	Fig. 23a Healthy gingiva	Fig. 23b Gingivitis	Fig. 23c Gingivitis	Fig. 23d Periodontitis
Gingival sulcus	Few bacteria in the sulcus	Plaque (P) along the gingival margin and in the gingival sulcus Leukocytes (L) beginning to accumulate beneath the plaque	Formation of sub-gingival plaque (Sgp)	Continued, apical penetration of the subgingival plaque
Sulcular epithelium Junctional epithelium	Thin epithelium displaying an even interface with the connective tissue Isolated leukocytes (L) within the epithelium	Formation of epithelial rete pegs in the connective tissue Infiltration of leukocytes adjacent to the plaque	Epithelial rete pegs more apically in the junctional epithelium Increased infiltration of leukocytes	Apical proliferation of the junctional epithelium along the root surface Isolated ulcerations
Connective tissue	Isolated inflammatory cells (Ic) in the connective tissue Few vascular loops (Vl) underneath the sulcular epithelium	Accumulation of inflammatory cells in the connective tissue Degradation of collagen fibers Vascular changes	Increase of inflammatory cells in the connective tissue Further degradation of collagen Increased vascular changes	Continued degradation of collagen fibers apically
Probing depth Periodontal pocket	Normal, 1-3-mm	Slight swelling of the gingiva and increased probing depth Pseudo-pocket	Increased swelling and deeper probing depth Pseudo-pocket	Deepened periodontal pocket
Alveolar bone				Resorption of the marginal alveolar bone (R)

Fig. 24. Gingivitis. Histological section. Plaque (P), red blood corpuscles (Rb), gingival exudate (Ge), inflammatory cells (Ic), blood vessels (Bv), decalcified enamel (De), dentin (D).

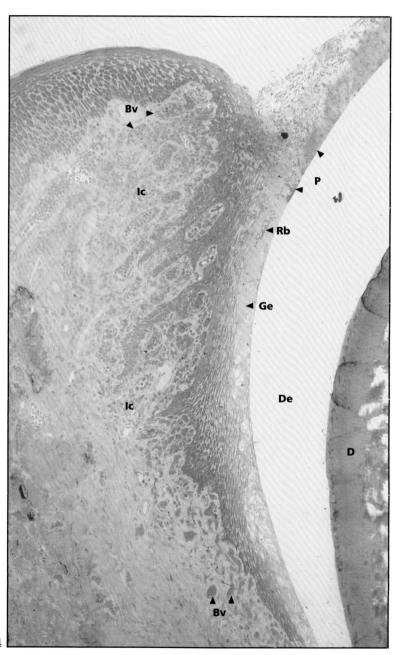

24

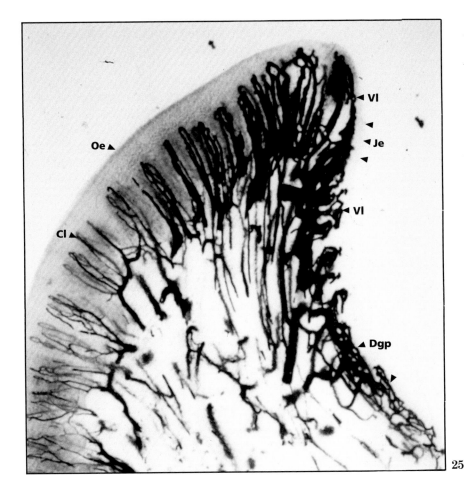

Fig 25. Gingivitis. Histological section demonstrating vascular proliferation. Oral epithelium (Oe), unstained junctional epithelium (Je), normal capillary loops underneath oral epithelium (Cl), vascular loops adjacent to sulcular/junctional epithelium (Vl), unchanged dentogingival plexus (Dgp).

Clinical signs of gingivitis

The redness of the gingiva intensifies in gingivitis and may eventually change to deep red or bluish red. The color changes usually begin in the papillae, spread along the gingival margin, and may finally affect the entire gingiva. The redness is caused by the increased vascular density in the connective tissue.

Color

The surface of the gingiva may become smooth and shiny due to the increased accumulation of tissue fluids. The stippling on the surface may dissappear due to the degradation of collagen.

Surface structure

Contour

Gingival swelling occurs initially at the gingival margin. Later, as the edema and vascular proliferation extends apically, it involves the entire gingiva.

Texture

The gingiva becomes spongy and loses its tonus due to collagen breakdown, edema and increased vascular density.

Probing depth

Increased probing depth may develop due to the gingival swelling, resulting in pseudo-pockets. This term means that the deepening is not related to loss of connective tissue attachment but to gingival swelling only.

Bleeding on probing

Gingivitis is characterized by an increased tendency to bleeding on gentle probing of the gingival sulcus or crevice.

Gingival Index

Clinical examination

Gingivitis can by detected by clinical examination. The various signs of gingivitis are evaluated: color, surface structure, contour, texture, probing depth and bleeding tendency. Most often, some of the signs are more apparent than others. The clinical appearance of gingivitis varies from one individual to another, and often also in various parts of the dentition within the same individual.

Gingival Index

Several different gingival index systems to express the degree of gingivitis have been developed and used clinically, particularly in scientific studies. In the Gingival Index according to Löe & Silness, the degree of gingivitis is evaluated for 4-6 aspects of each tooth and graded from 0 to 3. The Gingival Index for the individual patient is calculated by adding the scores for each examined surface and dividing this sum by the number of examined surfaces.

0 = clinically healthy gingiva, no inflammation;

1 = mild inflammation - slight change of color and contour - no bleeding on probing;

2 = moderate inflammation - redness and edema - bleeding on probing;

3 = severe inflammation - marked redness and edema - ulceration - spontaneous bleeding.

Bleeding scores

Bleeding on probing

Bleeding on probing is comparatively objective and easy to identify, and it may therefore be the most commonly used indicator for gingivitis. Healthy gingiva shows a limited tendency to bleed. The gingival crevice is probed with a thin but blunted periodontal probe, using a gentle probing force. Bleeding, visible within a few seconds, is generally a sign of gingival inflammation.

Bleeding scores

The presence or absence of bleeding on probing is recorded throughout the dentition. Commonly, bleeding gingiva is charted for six sites of each tooth: mesiobuccal, mid-buccal, distobuccal, mesiolingual, mid-lingual and distolingual. A percentage score is calculated for the patient by dividing the number of surfaces with bleeding by the total number of examined surfaces and multiplying by 100.

Prior to recording, the area under examination is dried using salivary evacuator, cotton rolls and compressed air. If saliva is present during examination, the bleeding will spread more easily along the gingival margin, and the site of origin for the bleeding will be more difficult to determine. Drying and preparation of one quadrant at a time is recommended.

Gingivitis

Questions

1. What is
   a) gingivitis?
   b) periodontitis?

2. What is the approximate time span for the development of gingivitis?

3. Gingivitis is reversible. Explain this statement.

4. What changes occur during the development of gingivitis
   a) in the sulcular/junctional epithelium?
   b) in the connective tissue?

5. What are the main types of inflammatory cells in gingivitis
   a) in the sulcular/junctional epithelium?
   b) in the connective tissue?

6. What types of vascular changes occur in gingivitis?

7. Which are the vascular alterations in gingivitis with respect to
   a) vascular topography?
   b) vascular permeability?
   c) vascular fragility?

8. What is spontaneous gingival bleeding?

9. What are the reasons for the increased bleeding tendency in gingivitis?

10. Describe the clinical characteristics of gingivitis with respect to
    a) color
    b) surface texture
    c) contour
    d) tonus
    e) probing depth
    f) bleeding on probing.

11. What is a pseudo-pocket?

12. Describe a gingival index.

13. What is the clinical significance of bleeding scores?

14. Describe the procedures to record bleeding scores in a patient.

Periodontitis

If left untreated, the inflammatory process in gingivitis may expand apically. Injury to the supporting structures of the teeth will ensue (periodontal ligament, cementum and alveolar bone). Periodontitis may develop.

Gingivitis leads to periodontitis

Many individuals do not develop periodontitis or are affected to a minor extent only, even though they may have gingivitis during an extended period of time. Other individuals may develop severe periodontitis, leading to the loss of teeth. Generally, periodontitis progresses slowly. In some individuals, however, the progression is more rapid. Most often, severe periodontal breakdown is not observed until the ages of 50-60 years, following 30-40 years of inflammatory involvement. Occasionally, however, severe periodontitis and loss of teeth may be seen at 25-30 years of age. The difference in susceptibility to periodontitis among various individuals may be explained by variations in immunological defense mechanisms, other host resistance factors and differences in the composition of the subgingival microbial flora (Fig. 29a-29e, p. 40; Fig. 30a-30d, p. 41).

Susceptibility to periodontitis

The composition of the gingival tissue changes due to the vascular, cellular and degenerative alterations. The coronal part of the junctional epithelium detaches from the tooth surface. The inflammatory process expands apically, accompanying the apical growth of the subgingival plaque. The connective tissue fibers immediately apical to the junctional epithelium are first degraded. In this way, the junctional epithelium can proliferate apically and onto the root surface. The continued apical shift of the junctional epithelium is coupled to the continued dissolution of collagen fibers inserted into the root. The marginal alveolar bone, also affected by the inflammatory process, starts to resorb.

Apical proliferation of the junctional epithelium

Bone resorption

Periodontal pocket

Increased bone loss

Increased tooth mobility

A periodontal pocket develops. The bottom of the probeable pocket approximates the level for the apical termination of the junctional epithelium (Fig. 23d, p. 30; Fig. 26). The resorption of the alveolar bone continues and the periodontal pocket deepens. The tooth support is increasingly compromised, leading to increased mobility of the teeth.

Fig 26. Periodontitis. Histological section. Altered junctional epithelium (Je) with epithelial rete pegs. The epithelium extends 1-2 mm apical to the cemento-enamel junction (Cej). The coronal cementum (C) has been scaled during previous treatment. Inflammatory cells (Ic) are seen infiltrating the connective tissue along the entire extent of the junctional epithelium. The height of the alveolar bone margin (Abm) may be somewhat reduced. An intraosseous defect has developed close to the root surface. During preparation of this section, the calculus (Ca) was detached and the soft tissues have undergone shrinkage and moved outward and downward, explaining the empty spaces between the gingiva and the root surface. Gingival groove (Gg), mucogingival junction (Mgj), alveolar mucosa (Am).

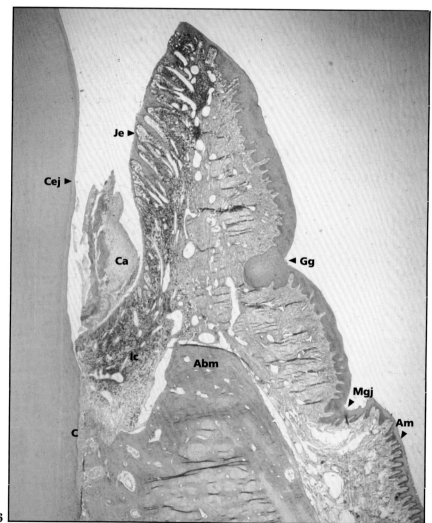

26

Recording probing depth

The probing depth, which is the distance between the gingival margin and the bottom of the probeable pocket, is measured to evaluate the magnitude of the periodontal deterioration (Fig. 27). The deepest probing depth for each tooth surface is recorded and charted following repeated probing ("searching").

A graduated periodontal probe is used. Six sites for each tooth are commonly charted: mesiobuccal, mid-buccal, distobuccal, mesiolingual, mid-lingual and distolingual. Charting of depths ≥4 mm only enhances the legibility of the records. Probing depths ≤3 mm could all be considered normal.

Several conditions may complicate the probing depth recordings: presence of calculus on the root surfaces (Fig. 28), aberrant root anatomy, dental restorations, oblique or irregular course of the coronal connective tissue attachment, bleeding during probing, limited access and visibility during probing and the patient pain threshold.

Searching for deepest probing depth

Complications during probing depth recordings

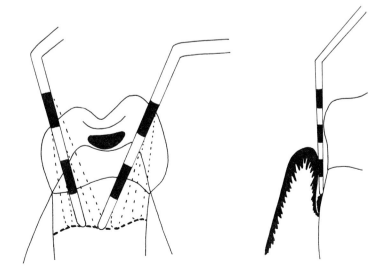

Fig. 27. During probing depth recordings, probing is repeated over each tooth surface ("searching"). The deepest measurement is recorded. Approximal surfaces should be probed from both buccal and lingual aspects to ensure that the entire surface has been explored.

Fig. 28. The probe may be stopped by subgingival calculus and an erroneous measurement will be obtained.

27, 28

Fig. 29a-29e. 45-year-old male with periodontitis. Gingival recession, primarily interdentally. Blueish (cyanotic), shiny, swollen (edematous) gingiva, particularly the papillae. Migration of the teeth has resulted in diastemas between the cuspid and the incisors on the right side (29a). Serumnal calculus, previously located subgingivally, is observed on the exposed palatal root surfaces (29b). The radiographs demonstrate reduced marginal bone height of varying degrees around the incisors, and presence of calculus on the approximal surfaces (29c-29e).

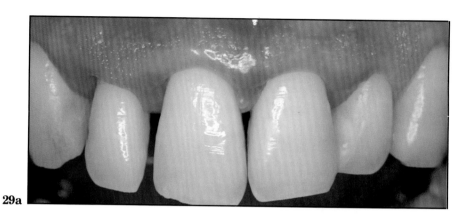

29a

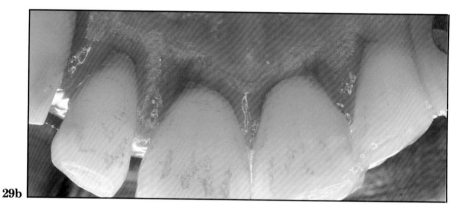

29b

29c, 29d, 29e

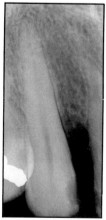
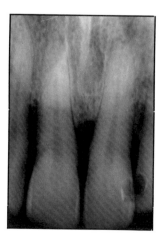
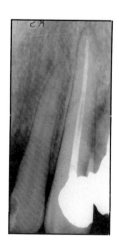

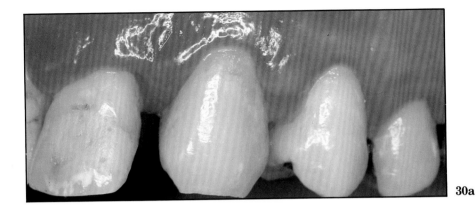

30a

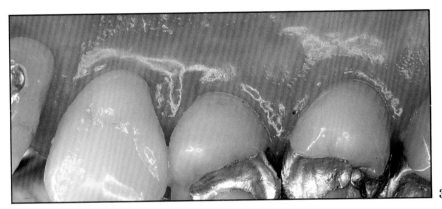

30b

Fig. 30a-30d. 28-year-old male with periodontitis. Red, shiny and swollen gingiva, especially for the buccal aspects of the cuspid and the lateral incisor (30a). Diastema between the lateral and the cuspid as a result of tooth migration. Plaque along the gingival margin on approximal and palatal surfaces (30b). The radiographs demonstrate bone loss for approximately half the root length of the lateral incisor (30c), as opposed to almost no bone loss for the 2nd premolar (30d).

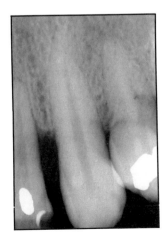 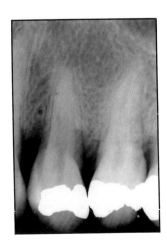

30c, 30d

Probing attachment level

The probing depths do not necessarily reflect the true loss of attachment for the teeth. Swelling of the gingiva in severe gingivitis may result in a deepened pocket without any loss of attachment at the cementoenamel junction (pseudo-pocket). Conversely, due to gingival recession, the probing depths may still be shallow in spite of substantial loss of attachment (Fig. 31, 32a).

Fig. 31. Three illustrations (A, B and C) showing loss of attachment amounting to 2 mm (A), 4 mm (B) and 6 mm (C). For all three situations, the probing depth is 4 mm due to the differences in the location of the gingival margin.

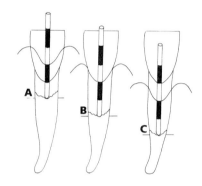

31

The distance from the cementoenamel junction to the depth of the probeable pocket should be recorded if a proper measurement of loss of tooth support is required. This measurement is termed probing attachment level or clinical attachment level (Fig. 32a, 32b).

Fig. 32a, 32b. Two situations, both with probing attachment loss amounting to 6 mm. Probing depth in Fig. 32a = 4.5 mm and in Fig. 32b = 9 mm.

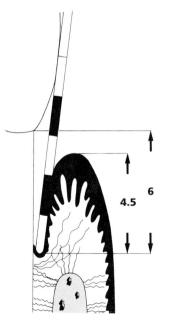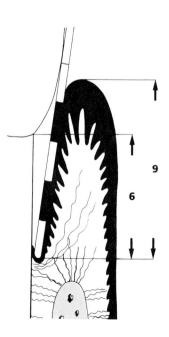

32a, 32b

Periodontitis

Questions

1. Define periodontitis.

2. Why do not all cases of gingivitis gradually develop into periodontitis?

3. Describe the development of periodontal pockets.

4. Describe the procedures for measurement and charting of probing depths.

5. Name some of the factors complicating probing depth measurement.

6. What is the significance of probing attachment levels?

Gingival suppuration

Cellular exudate

In gingival health, minute amounts of exudate of fluids and inflammatory cells ooze into the gingival sulcus. In gingivitis and periodontitis, the exudation intensifies. Plaque at the gingival margin and subgingivally may block the drainage of emigrated inflammatory cells and shedded epithelial cells from the junctional epithelium. This leads to cellular accumulation between the subgingival plaque and the junctional epithelium. If drainage is facilitated, such as by opening the periodontal pocket with a probe, this accumulation may be discharged together with tissue fluids and microorganisms. A droplet of pus becomes visible at the gingival margin. Occasionally, in case of voluminous accumulation, spontaneous discharge may occur (Fig. 33, p. 45).

Accumulation of tissue fluids, cells and microorganisms

The gradual drainage of the cellular exudate is perhaps most inhibited in deep pockets and in pockets with calculus. Pus is therefore more likely to be observed in deeper pockets. The amounts of pus may vary from a barely visible droplet to extensive amounts. Large overhangs on dental restorations may also contribute to impeded drainage and visible suppuration.

Identification of gingival pus

To identify gingival pus, the area under examination is first dried. A periodontal probe is inserted into the periodontal pocket. The pocket orifice is widened by angling the probe away from the tooth, followed by gentle retraction of the probe tip and careful inspection (Fig. 34-35, p. 45). The presence of pus may often be overlooked due to simultaneous bleeding, which disguises the suppuration. It is sometimes difficult to distinguish pus from voluminous dental plaque in the pocket orifice due to the similarity of color and consistency.

Unpleasant taste

Not infrequently, patients may suspect suppuration because of an unpleasant taste.

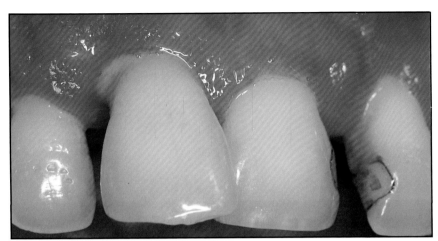

Fig. 33. Accumulation of pus along the gingival margin at the distobuccal aspect of right central incisor and to a lesser extent at the distobuccal aspect of the left central incisor and the buccal aspect of the left lateral incisor. Migration of the teeth has resulted in both "crowding" and diastemas.

33

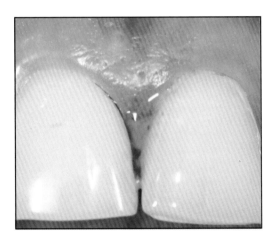 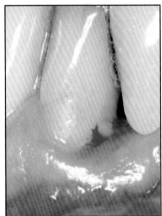

Fig. 34, 35. Droplets of pus and blood seen after examination using a periodontal probe.

34, 35

Gingival suppuration

Questions

1. Describe the events leading to the accumulation of pus in periodontal pockets.

2. What are the components of gingival pus?

3. Describe the procedures for detection of gingival pus.

Tooth migration

In individuals with advanced periodontitis and severe loss of supporting tissues, one or more teeth may gradually move from their original positions in the dental arch. Maxillary incisors tend to spread buccally, resulting in an increased horizontal overlap and in the formation of diastemata. The migration is probably explained by the fact that the diminished tooth support no longer can withstand forces from tongue thrust, from opposing and neighboring teeth during mastication and bruxism and from habitual activities of various kinds, such as pipe smoking.

It has been suggested that inflamed gingival tissues also may exert pressure. The various forces affecting the teeth may gradually change the position of compromised teeth in the dental arch. Diastema, crowding, rotation, tipping and elongation may be signs of tooth migration in advanced periodontitis (Fig. 29a-29e, p. 40; Fig. 30a-30d, p. 41; Fig. 33, p. 45; Fig. 36a, 36b).

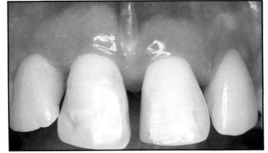

36a

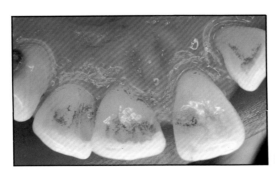

36b

Fig. 36a, 36b. 48-year-old woman with advanced periodontitis and tooth migration. According to the patient, a small gap was always present between the central incisors. Note the limited signs of gingival inflammation in this case.

Tooth migration

Questions

1. What are the reasons for tooth migration in periodontitis?

2. Describe various changes in tooth position that may develop due to migration of teeth in periodontitis.

Tooth mobility

Teeth normally show some mobility, although minute. The wavy arrangement of the collagen fibers in the periodontal ligament permits the teeth to move within the alveolus. This is termed physiological tooth mobility. Studies using special instruments to record tooth mobility have shown that physiological tooth mobility varies between different teeth due to differences in root anatomy and associated differences in anchorage. Single-rooted teeth with short roots have somewhat higher physiological tooth mobility than teeth with long and sturdy roots, such as cuspids and multi-rooted teeth.

Physiological tooth mobility

A tooth that is repeatedly exposed to large forces, such as those from interfering tooth contacts during mastication or bruxism (traumatic occlusion) or from forces during orthodontic treatment, may develop increased mobility. Parts of the bony wall of the alveolus resorb and remodel, and the width of the periodontal ligament increases. The position of the tooth may change somewhat, thereby compensating for the traumatic influence. The tooth also acquires increased mobility. Radiographically, increased tooth mobility can often be observed from the presence of a widened periodontal ligament, particularly in the apical parts of the root (Fig. 37c, p. 50). In some cases, the traumatic forces may be spontaneously eliminated due to compensatory tooth movement. More often, occlusal adjustment by a professional is required to achieve healing of the periodontal ligament and normalization of the tooth mobility.

Traumatic forces

Increased width of the periodontal ligament

Due to the loss of tooth support in periodontitis, tooth mobility may increase. The degree of increased mobility is related not only to the loss of alveolar bone but also to various traumatic forces and to the degree of inflammation of the gingiva. The pathological tooth mobility in periodontitis can be reduced following treatment and elimination of the gingival inflammation.

Pathological tooth mobility in periodontitis

Quantity and quality of remaining periodontal tissues

Thus, it is not only the amount of remaining tooth support that governs the degree of stability of a tooth but also the quality of the remaining tissues. A tooth with comparatively little support but with healthy tissues may be more stable than a tooth with quite ample support but with inflamed tissues.

Recording tooth mobility

Increased tooth mobility is detected and recorded by exposing the tooth to a moderate force using a suitable instrument (Fig. 37a, 37b). Horizontal tooth mobility is evaluated following application of a force in a buccolingual direction. The amplitude of the displacement of the incisal edge or the cusp is estimated in mm. In severe periodontitis, increased mobility in the vertical (longitudinal) direction may also occur and is recorded following application of a force in an apical direction. Increased tooth mobility is commonly rated as follows:

Horizontal mobility

Vertical mobility

- grade 1: horizontal mobility <1 mm
- grade 2: horizontal mobility ≥1 mm
- grade 3: vertical mobility.

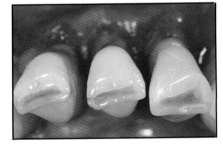

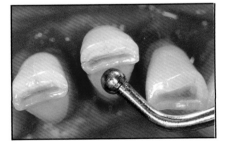

37a

Fig. 37a-37c. A slight force from the lingual aspect resulted in displacement of the incisal egde >1 mm - mobility grade 2 (37a, 37b). The radiograph shows advanced bone loss and widened periodontal ligaments for the central incisors (37c).

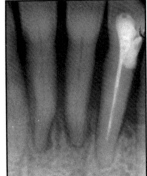

37c, 37b

Tooth mobility

Questions

1. What is physiological tooth mobility?

2. Describe conditions that may lead to increased tooth mobility.

3. What are the tissue changes explaining the radiographic observation of a widened periodontal ligament?

4. What are the causes of increased tooth mobility in periodontitis?

5. Describe the clinical procedures for identifying increased tooth mobility.

6. Describe a system for classifying increased tooth mobility.

Gingival recession

Gingival recession means that the gingival margin has migrated apically and that the root surface has become exposed. The recession can be localized to an individual surface of a single tooth or involve a multitude of surfaces and teeth in the dentition.

Fig. 38a-38e. 36-year-old male with advanced periodontitis. Gingival recession interdentally between the central and lateral incisors on both sides (38a). Additional recession taking place after oral hygiene instruction and subgingival debridement of the teeth (38b). Bone loss amounting to about half of the root length (38c-38e).

38a

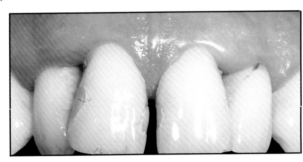

38b

38c, 38d, 38e

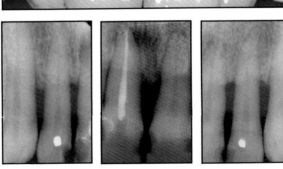

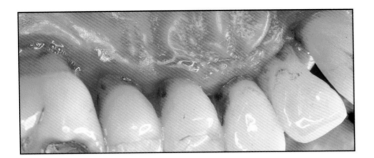

39a

Fig. 39a, 39b. 42-year-old man with advanced periodontitis and generalized gingival recession. Calculus, previously located subgingivally, has become exposed due to the recession (39a). Some additional recession occurred after oral hygiene instruction and debridement (39b). The interdental gingiva continues to exhibit signs of inflammation.

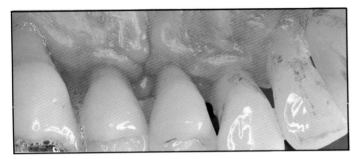

39b

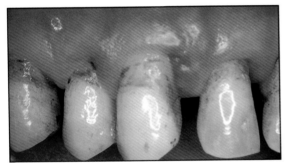 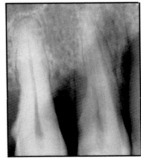

Fig. 40a-40d. 41-year-old man with periodontitis and gingival recession. The exposed root surfaces show spots of serumal calculus (40a). The radiographs reveal varying bone loss (40c, 40d). Additional recession following oral hygiene instruction and debridement (40b).

40a, 40c

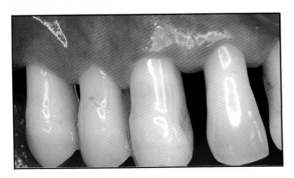 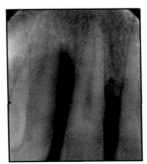

40b, 40d

Localized gingival recession

Localized gingival recession can often be observed for teeth positioned facially in the dental arch, such as buccal surfaces of maxillary cuspids. Corresponding recession for lingually positioned teeth may also occur, such as the palatal surfaces of maxillary molars. A thin plate of alveolar bone or a dehiscence of the bone (Fig. 11b, p. 15) combined with a thin gingiva may predispose to gingival recession in these situations.

Generalized gingival recession

Due to periodontitis

In periodontitis, either localized or generalized gingival recession is common. The inflammatory process, initiated and maintained by microorganisms, degrades the gingival connective tissue and alveolar bone. The gingival margin migrates apically and the roots are gradually exposed. The patients frequently observe this, remarking that their teeth have become "long".

Due to treatment

Gingival recession usually occurs following treatment of periodontitis with oral hygiene instruction and debridement. The amount of recession that takes place depends on several conditions: the degree of pre-treatment edema and vascularization of the gingiva, the pocket depths, the amount and type of alveolar bone loss and the anatomy of the teeth and the alveolar bone. When the inflammation of the gingiva is eliminated, the gingival margin recedes to a more apical position (Fig. 38a-38e, p. 52; Fig. 40a-40d, p. 53; Fig. 41a-41c, p. 56). Surgical treatment also leads to gingival recession, particularly if gingival tissues have been removed, as in gingivectomy.

The final outcome of treatment in terms of gingival recession, however, bears little relationship to the method of treatment: debridement without a surgical procedure, with gingivectomy or with periodontal flap surgery. The long-term position of the gingival margin is related to the remaining height of the alveolar bone, the anatomy of the teeth and their position in the alveolar process.

Localized gingival recession can sometimes be observed associated with a vestibular frenulum attached close to the gingival margin. During movements of the lips and cheek, the connective tissue fibers of such a frenulum may cause a pull to the marginal gingiva. The closeness of the frenulum to the gingival margin may also interfere with toothbrushing in the area. Tissue trauma and inflammation may lead to gingival recession for the tooth adjacent to the frenulum (Fig. 42-44, p. 57).

Due to interfering frenulum

Individuals using snuff (smokeless tobacco) often develop mucosal and gingival lesions in the area where the snuff is placed. The degree of injury is related to the frequency of snuff usage. Epithelial erosions develop due to the caustic effect of the alkaline snuff (pH = 8-9). A white-yellow lesion with a wrinkled surface may develop, sometimes combined with a localized gingival recession. The thickness of the epithelium increases, and its surface displays hyperkeratinization (Fig. 45, p. 57). An inflammatory reaction develops in the connective tissue, leading to tissue degradation.

Due to snuff

Gingival recession may also be caused by overzealous toothbrushing (Fig. 46a, 46b, p. 57) (see separate section, pp. 59-63).

Due to trauma from toothbrushing

A certain amount of gingival recession may be inevitable in some individuals in spite of continuously healthy gingival conditions and gentle toothbrushing: that is, gingival recession may be a normal, age-related alteration. Lack of facial or lingual bone over the root and a thin gingiva may be a prerequisite for such alterations.

Age-related gingival recession?

Fig. 41a-41c. 55-year-old woman prior to treatment (41a), 9 months after oral hygiene instruction and debridement (41b) and 4 years later without additional treatment (41c). Gradual gingival recession coupled with improved appearance of the gingiva.

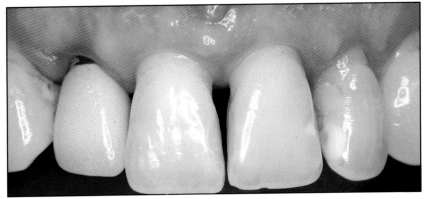

41a

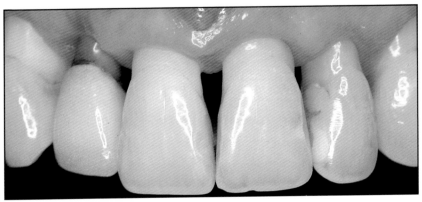

41b

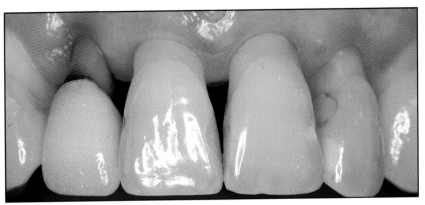

41c

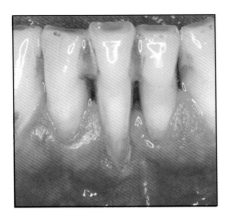
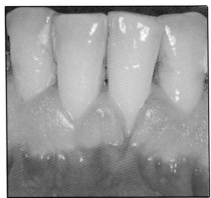

42, 43

Fig. 42, 43. Gingival recession associated with a vestibular frenulum. The closeness of the frenulum to the gingival margin may interfere with the toothbrushing.

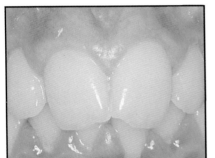
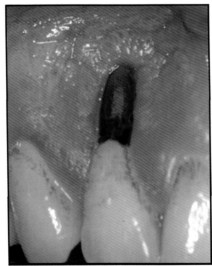

44, 45

Fig. 44. 12-year-old girl with gingival recession at the mandibular left lateral incisor, possibly as an effect of the closeness of the frenulum attachment combined with gingival inflammation. Note the inflamed gingival papillae in the maxilla.

Fig. 45. Extensive gingival recession and marked discoloration of the root surface casued by placement of snuff in this area. Hyperkeratinization of the gingiva.

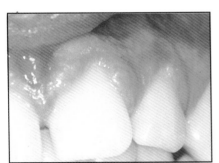
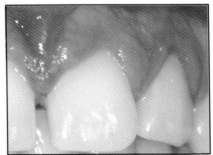

46a, 46b

Fig. 46a, 46b. 15-year-old boy with gingival recession in central and lateral incisors following overzealous toothbrushing (46a). The marginal gingiva has partly regained its location following two weeks of more gentle toothbrushing (46b).

Gingival recession

Questions

1. Define gingival recession.

2. Name the reasons for gingival recession.

3. What are the mechanisms for the development of gingival recession
   a) in periodontitis?
   b) due to interfering frenulum?
   c) after periodontal treatment?
   d) following the use of snuff?

Oral hygiene lesions

Improper oral hygiene routines may lead to lesions of the gingiva and the teeth. The lesions may become permanent but do generally not jeopardize the longevity of the teeth. Identification of these traumatic injuries should be part of periodontal examination.

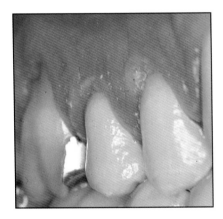
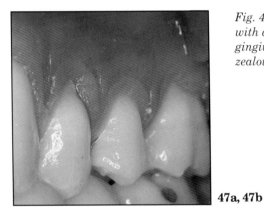

Fig. 47a, 47b. 20-year-old man with a multitude of buccal gingival recessions due to overzealous toothbrushing.

47a, 47b

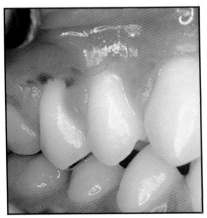
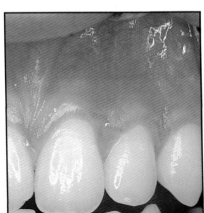

Fig. 48a, 48b. 14-year-old boy with excessive gingival lesions due to overzealous toothbrushing. Gingival recession and ulceration in right premolars and cuspid (48a) and in left central and lateral incisors (48b).

48a, 48b

Buccal and lingual gingival lesions

Erosion

A superficial epithelial lesion, an erosion, can develop following vigorous toothbrushing, particularly following the use of a hard or a new toothbrush. The erosions may occur at the gingival margin or more apically on the attached gingiva. They are characterized by the peeled, red appearance of the epithelium (Fig. 49, p. 62). More forceful trauma may cause a removal of the entire epithelium - ulceration (Fig. 48a, 48b, p. 59; Fig. 50, p. 62).

Ulceration

Hyperkeratinization

In some patients, an increased keratinization of the epithelial surface can be observed. Hyperkeratinization gives the surface a white color tone and is probably the result of repeated, limited injuries over a long period of time (Fig. 53, 54, p. 62).

Fissure

A vertical fissure of the gingival margin is a comparatively common lesion following overly vigorous toothbrushing. This lesion may develop following repeated trauma to the marginal gingiva. When observed, the fissure may be combined with erosion of the epithelial surface (Fig. 53, 54, p. 62).

Recession

Gingival recession as a result of excessive toothbrushing is primarily observed for buccal roots of teeth positioned more buccally in the dental arch than the adjacent teeth. Buccal bone may be missing over these roots, facilitating the progression of the recession (Fig. 11b, p. 15). Corresponding conditions may manifest over lingually displaced teeth and roots, such as the palatal roots of maxillary molars. However, gingival recession due to overzealous toothbrushing may also unfold over roots of well-aligned teeth (Fig. 46a, 46b, p. 57; Fig. 47a, 47b, p. 59).

U-shape

V-shape

Localized gingival recession may extend over the entire width of the tooth and then takes a U-shape. Narrower recessions are generally V-shaped (Fig. 54, p. 62).

Hyperplasia

An increased thickness of the gingiva, hyperplasia, may also result from excessive toothbrushing (Fig. 53, 54, p. 62).

Interdental gingival lesions

Incorrect use of toothpicks and interdental brushes may result in epithelial erosions or ulcerations of the interdental papillae.

Erosion
Ulceration

Triangular tooth-cleaning sticks, used upside down, may lead to a fissure in the papillary area. Similar injuries can be created after improper use of dental floss (Fig. 51, p. 62).

Fissure

Buccal and lingual dental defects

Wedge-shaped defects in the cervical portion of the teeth occur primarily for buccal surfaces. Following initial gingival recession, loss of tooth structure emerges immediately apical to the cementoenamel junction. The wedge-shaped defects develop due to forceful brushing with scrubbing movements in combination with the use of a toothpaste with abrasives (Fig. 52, p. 62).

Wedge-shaped cervical defects

Approximal dental defects

Occasionally, loss of tooth substance may be observed for approximal surfaces, such as after frequent use of interdental cleaning sticks in combination with an abrasive dentifrice.

Toxic and allergic lesions

Oral rinses with the antiseptic chlorhexidine may sporadically lead to epithelial erosions of the gingiva or the oral mucosa due to a toxic mechanism.

Toxic reactions

On rare occasions, allergic reactions to components of toothpastes may arise, manifesting with erythema and erosion of the gingiva or the oral mucosa.

Allergic reactions

49, 50

Fig. 49. Example of a common type of minor epithelial erosion, located on the buccal gingiva of the lateral incisor.

Fig. 50. Extensive erosion and ulceration of the gingiva following overzealous toothbrushing.

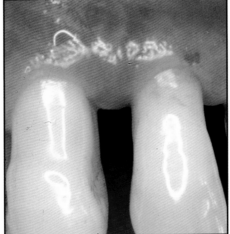

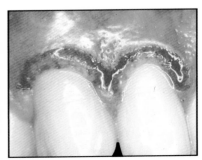

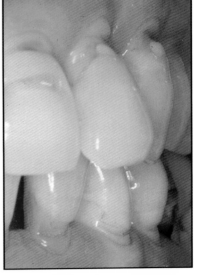

Fig. 51. Ulcerations interdentally and palatally following the improper use of dental floss.

Fig. 52. Deep wedge-shaped, cervical defects on maxillary and mandibular teeth.

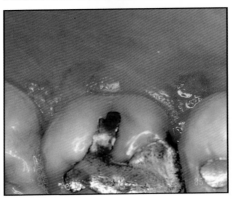

51, 52

Fig. 53. Exceptionally deep fissure on the buccal gingiva of the 1st molar. Note a small fissure in the 2nd premolar. Gingival hyperplasia and hyperkeratinization are also evident.

Fig. 54. Gingival recession, fissure, hyperplasia and hyperkeratinization of the cuspid.

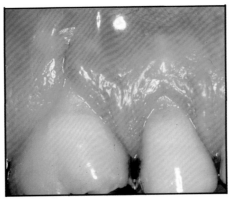

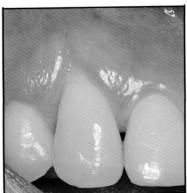

53, 54

Oral hygiene lesions

Questions

1. What different types of lesions may develop following overzealous oral hygiene procedures
   a) in the gingiva?
   b) in the teeth?

2. What is epithelial erosion and how does it arise?

3. What is epithelial hyperkeratinization and how does it develop?

4. Describe the appearance of fissures at the gingival margin caused by traumatic toothbrushing and how they may originate.

5. List the typical locations at which gingival recession occurs as a result of excessive toothbrushing. Why?

6. Describe the variations in the shape of localized gingival recession caused by traumatic toothbrushing.

7. What types of interdental gingival lesions arise because of improper oral hygiene procedures and how do they originate?

8. Describe the appearance of dental defects with loss of tooth structure following overzealous oral hygiene procedures.

9. What circumstances lead to cervical, wedge-shaped defects?

10. Give some examples of toxic or allergic reactions of the gingiva or the mucosa related to oral hygiene.

Alveolar bone changes

Rate of progression

The rate of alveolar bone loss in periodontitis often varies for different parts of the dentition and also for different aspects of individual teeth. Thus, the alveolar bone margin often exhibits an uneven course throughout the dentition. The reasons for the variation in the rate of progression are not fully understood. However, sites prone to plaque accumulation tend to show an increased progression rate. Approximal surfaces generally display more plaque and subgingival calculus, and they also show more bone loss and deeper pockets than other surfaces of the teeth. Other conditions that may enhance plaque retention and progression of periodontitis are overhanging restorations, furcation involvement, concavities and furrows on the roots.

Horizontal bone loss

A similar rate of bone loss for adjacent teeth in the dentition results in an even level of the reduced alveolar bone crest and is termed horizontal bone loss (Fig. 55, 56).

Fig. 55. Mandibular incisors with normal bone height. The anatomical distance between the cemento-enamel junction and the bone crest is normally 1-1.5 mm. In radiographs, it may vary more due to the limitation of radiographs in revealing thin crestal bone, and due to variations in X-ray projection.

Fig. 56. Horizontal bone loss exceeding half of the normal bone height. The conical root shape implies that the tooth supporting area is reduced even more. Left central incisor shows a widened periodontal ligament - evidence of increased tooth mobility.

55, 56

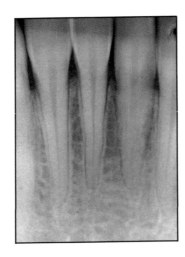 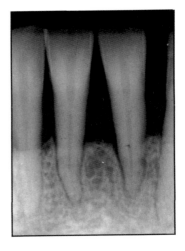

Intraosseous defects

An increased rate of bone loss for one or two surfaces of a tooth compared with the other surfaces of this same tooth results in the formation of a localized defect in the alveolar bone. Such defects are termed intraosseous, infrabony or vertical defects (Fig. 57a-57d; Fig. 61a-61c, 62, p. 68).

Vertical bone loss

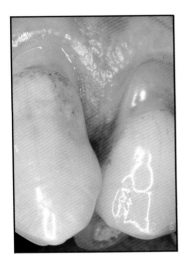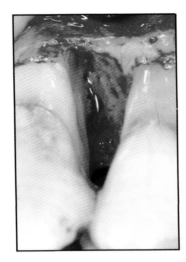

Fig. 57a-57d. Intraosseous defect at the distal aspect of the cuspid, prior to (57a) and after flap elevation and soft tissue curettage (57b). Apically, the defect has three osseous walls (palatal, distal and buccal). More coronal, only a distal wall is present. The buccal and palatal walls can be discerned in the radiographs (57c, 57d).

57a, 57b

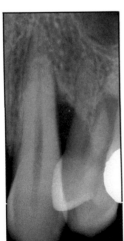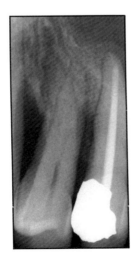

57c, 57d

In the presence of a narrow intraosseous defect, such as a defect related to a root furrow, the probing depth will be increased only for a very limited portion of the circumference of the tooth. A radiograph of the area may not disclose any bone loss, as the bone density of adjacent structures may overshadow the defect. For detection, the radiographic examination needs to be combined with probing depth measurements. This example reinforces why probing depth measurements need to be performed carefully and at a number of locations around the tooth. A comparison of the recorded probing depths and the radiographic image will help to clarify the nature of the defect.

1-, 2- or 3-wall intraosseous defects

Intraosseous defects are commonly classified into 1-, 2- or 3-wall defects, depending on the number of available osseous walls bordering the defect.
- 3-wall defect: bordered by 3 osseous walls and 1 wall formed by the root surface (Fig. 58a, p. 67).
- 2-wall defect: bordered by 2 osseous walls, 1 root wall and 1 wall formed by gingival soft tissue (Fig. 58b, p. 67).
- 1-wall defect: bordered by 1 osseous wall, 1 root wall and 2 soft tissue walls (Fig. 58c, p. 67).

Combination defect

Intraosseous defects usually consist of a combination of the above basic types. The coronal part may have 1 wall, the middle part 2 walls and the apical part 3 walls (Fig. 57a-57d, p. 65; Fig. 61a-61c, 62, p. 68).

Interdental crater

Defects between two adjacent teeth bordered by the two approximal root surfaces and buccal and lingual bone are termed interdental craters.

Classification of intraosseous defects has been introduced because of the assumption that regenerative periodontal therapy aiming at bone fill of the defects may be more successful in defects with more osseous walls.

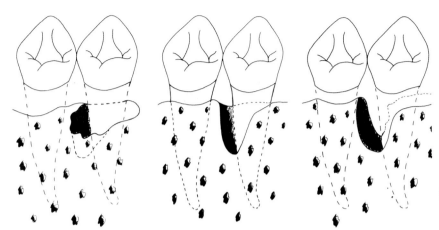

58a, 58b, 58c

The nature of an intraosseous defect cannot be determined from radiographs alone, although experienced clinicians often acquire a fairly accurate perception. Comparison with the probing depths will facilitate the determination.

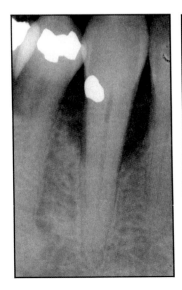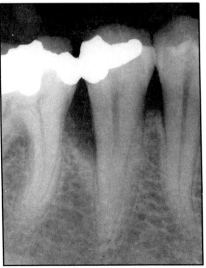

Fig. 59. Intraosseous defects for the mesial and distal aspects, and probably also for the lingual aspect of the cuspid. For the mesial surface, the appearance suggests a 1-wall defect, possibly with 2 or 3 walls in the apical part. For the distal surface, the radiograph indicates a 2-wall defect. The lingual (buccal?) bone margin appears to be at the same level as the fundus of the mesial and distal defects.

Fig. 60. 2-wall intraosseous defect at the distal aspect of the 2nd premolar. A 3rd wall is probably present more apically.

59, 60

61a

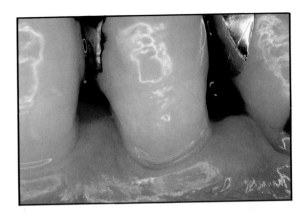

Fig. 61a-61c. Intraosseous defects at the mesial aspects of the 2nd premolar and the 1st molar, prior to (61a) and after flap elevation and soft tissue curettage (61b). The defect for the mesial surface of the 2nd premolar has a lingual and a mesial bone wall, and possibly also a small buccal wall apically (2-wall defect, possibly with an apical 3-wall component). The defect on the mesial surface of the 1st molar also has a lingual and a mesial osseous wall, but a higher buccal wall. Radiographically, the contours of the lingual and buccal walls can be discerned (61c).

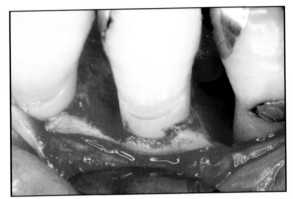

61b

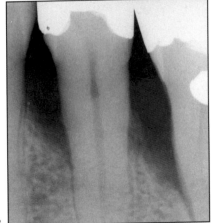

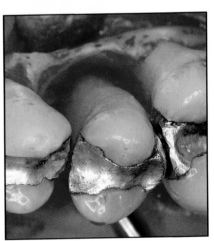

Fig. 62. Circumferential intraosseous defect at the buccal aspect of the 2nd premolar. This defect type cannot be classified according to the conventional 1-, 2- and 3-wall system.

61c, 62

Furcation involvement

Progression of periodontitis in multi-rooted teeth extends the inflammatory process to the furcation areas between the roots. The clinical term furcation involvement is used to denote periodontal breakdown and pocket formation reaching to or beyond the furcation apertures. Once furcation involvement has been established, the progression continues not only apically but also horizontally (Fig. 63a, 63b).

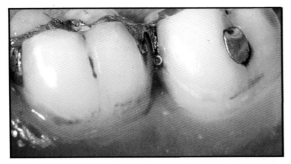

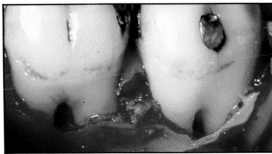

Fig. 63a, 63b. Buccal furcation involvement of mandibular 1st and 2nd molars, prior to (63a) and after flap elevation and soft tissue curettage (63b). For both defects, the horizontal probing depth amounts to 3-4 mm (class 2 involvement).

63a

63b

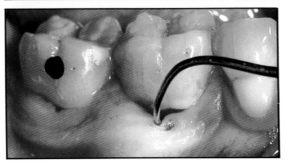

Fig. 64. Buccal furcation involvement of mandibular 1st molar identified with a furcation probe.

64

Bifurcation involvement Trifurcation involvement

Clinical inspection and probing

Furcation involvement may occur for maxillary and mandibular molars, first maxillary premolars and occasionally in normally single-rooted teeth. In 2-rooted teeth, the term bifurcation involvement is often used. In 3-rooted teeth, the expression trifurcation involvement may be applied.

Recording of furcation involvement

Furcation involvement is identified by clinical inspection and probing, combined with radiographic evaluation. A straight periodontal probe may be used. Often, however, the probing is facilitated by the use of specially designed furcation probes or by the use of a periodontal curette. To detect involvement, the probe tip is moved against the root surface towards the presumed location of the furcation aperture (Fig. 64, p. 69; Fig. 67a-67f, p. 71). If possible, both roots of the furcation should be probed. Buccal and lingual furcation involvement of mandibular molars, and buccal involvement of maxillary molars are usually not difficult to identify. However, finding and grading involvement for maxillary approximal furcations may be more difficult, due to the limited access caused by the neighboring teeth. These involvements are usually best detected and recorded from the palatal aspect. Again, clinical inspection and probing should be supplemented with radiographic observation (Fig. 66; Fig. 67a-67f, p. 71).

Fig. 65. Furcation involvements of maxillary 1st and 2nd molars (same teeth as in Fig. 64). The involvement for the 2nd molar can be observed radiographically. For the 1st molar, the involvement is masked by a thick buccal ledge of alveolar bone.

Fig. 66. Furcation involvement between the buccal roots of maxillary 1st molar. An osseous contour extending distally from the furcation center suggests that the furcation center may also be reached from the distal aspect (between the distobuccal and palatal roots). The radiograph provides little guidance as to any furcation involvement from the mesial aspect. (see Fig. 67a-67f, p. 71).

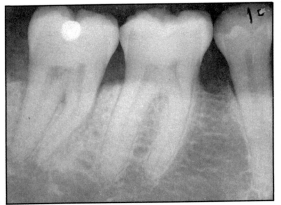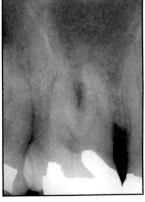

65, 66

67a, 67b

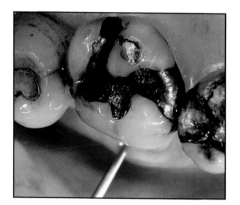
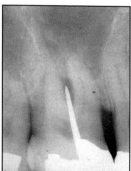

Fig. 67a-67f. Approaches for probing furcation involvements of buccal (67a ,67b), mesial (67c, 67d) and distal (67e, 67f) aspects of a maxillary 1st molar (same tooth as in Fig. 66). Radiographs with the probe in place demonstrate that the furcation can be reached from all 3 aspects (class 3 involvement). The mesial osseous contour sloping into the furcation can best be observed in Fig. 67f, whilst the distal bone contour is best seen in Fig. 67b. The probing from the distal aspect is performed with a furcation probe.

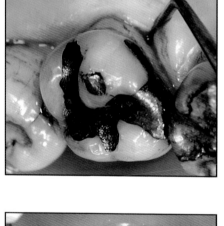
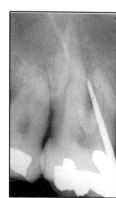

67c, 67d

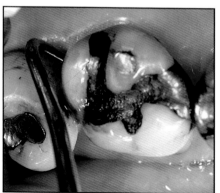
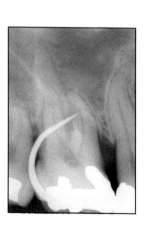

67e, 67f

Radiographic evaluation

Following more substantial loss of bone in the furcation area, the involvement can usually be observed radiographically (Fig. 71a, 71b, 72a, 72b, p. 74). Remaining bone in the furcation area, however, may disguise the involvement and lead to erroneous interpretation (Fig. 65, p. 70). Approximal involvement in the maxilla can often be difficult to detect due to superimposition of other radiopaque structures. Radiographic examination, therefore, cannot substitute for clinical examination but constitutes a useful supplement. However, a radiograph may disclose a furcation involvement that is difficult to observe clinically due to limited access. Both methods of examination are advised.

The degree of furcation involvement is commonly graded as follows:

Class 1 involvement

Class 1: initial involvement. The furcation aperture can be felt during probing. The horizontal probing depth is less than one third of the entire furcation depth. Radiographically, little or no bone loss may be observed (Fig. 68a).

Class 2 involvement

Class 2: partial involvement. The horizontal probing depth is one third or more of the total furcation depth, but the furcation cannot be probed through-and-through. Radiographically, bone loss is commonly seen (Fig. 68b).

Fig. 68a-68c. Illustration of furcation involvement class 1 (68a), class 2 (68b) and class 3 (68c).

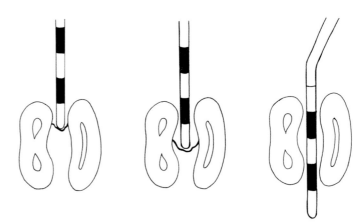

68a, 68b, 68c

Class 3: through-and-through involvement. The probe passes through the entire horizontal dimension of the furcation, from one aspect to the opposite aspect of the tooth. Radiographically, bone loss is usually apparent (Fig. 68c, p. 72; Fig. 70a, 70b, 71a, 71b, 72a, 72b, p. 74).

Class 3 involvement

Classification of the degree of furcation involvement is often difficult and includes a definite subjective component of evaluation. Following examination, the degree of involvement should be charted for each furcation area.

Routine examination of furcation involvement is an important part of periodontal examination. Early detection may facilitate the therapeutic attempts to prevent or retard continuous progression. At an early stage, both debridement by a professional and routine oral hygiene procedures by the patient may be effective. At later stages, furcation areas may be difficult or impossible to clean. Root amputation is occasionally performed to eradicate the furcation problem.

Early diagnosis

Early diagnosis of furcation involvement is thus important in the efforts to improve the longevity of these teeth, known to have a less favorable prognosis than teeth without furcation involvement (Fig. 69a, 69b).

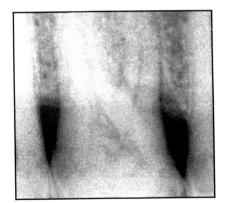 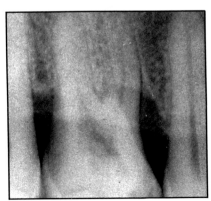

Fig. 69a, 69b. Furcation involvement of maxillary 1st molar. In this case, the involvement is less obvious from the X-ray projection used for the bite-wing film (69a), and more noticeable from the projection used for the periapical film (69b).

69a, 69b

Fig. 70a, 70b. Class 3 furcation involvement of mandibular 1st molar, from the buccal (70a) and lingual (70b) aspects.

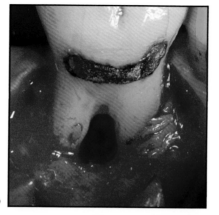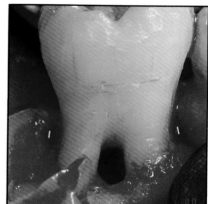

70a, 70b

Fig. 71a, 71b. Class 3 furcation involvement of mandibular 1st molar. The radiograph (71b) shows two osseous contours over the tooth, one buccal and one lingual. Comparison of the level of the buccal crest of bone in Fig. 71a with the two contours in the radiograph suggests that the buccal crest is more coronal than the lingual crest.

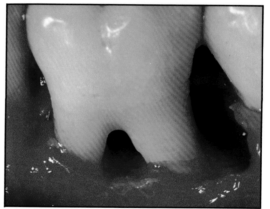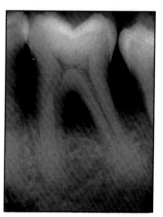

71a, 71b

Fig. 72a, 72b. Class 3 furcation involvement of mandibular 1st molar.

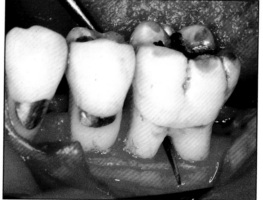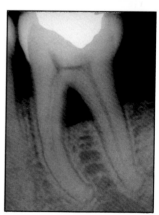

72a, 72b

Alveolar bone changes

Questions

1. What are the general patterns of bone loss in periodontitis?

2. Identify some conditions that may affect the rate of progression in periodontitis.

3. Define
   a) intraosseous defect
   b) interdental crater.

4. What other terms are used to denote an intraosseous defect?

5. How is a localized intraosseous defect best discovered in a patient?

6. Describe
   a) a 1-wall defect
   b) a 2-wall defect
   c) a 3-wall defect
   d) a combination defect.

7. Define the term furcation involvement.

8. Which teeth in the dentition may exhibit
   a) bifurcation involvement?
   b) trifurcation involvement?

9. How is furcation involvement best discovered in a patient?

10. Describe the clinical identification of furcation involvement
    a) class 1
    b) class 2
    c) class 3.

11. Describe the approximate radiographic characteristics of furcation involvement
    a) class 1
    b) class 2
    c) class 3.

12. Describe some of the limitations involved in the clinical and radiographic identification of furcation involvement.

Radiographic evaluation

Periapical radiographs

Bite-wing radiographs

Panoramic radiographs

Radiographic examination is required to evaluate the extent of periodontal breakdown throughout the dentition and to establish a proper treatment plan. An entire set of radiographs is usually necessary to detect possible variation in bone morphology throughout the mouth. Periapical films supplemented with bite-wing films are commonly used, as this combination is useful for diagnosis of both caries and periodontal disease. Panoramic radiographs, coupled with intraoral films for detailed analysis, may also be used. In cases of gingivitis with little suspicion of underlying periodontitis, a set of bite-wing films may suffice. Supplementary films can be obtained if required, based on the clinical and radiographic observations.

Proper projection

The X-ray projection during examination should be perpendicular to the dental arch, providing images of the interdental bone with minimal superimposition of the roots. Some standardization of the radiographic techniques in clinical practice may be useful, as this will facilitate the comparison of radiographs obtained at different time points.

Fig. 73, 74. Two radiographs of the same mandibular incisor area showing differences in the image of the bone support for the distal aspect of the left central incisor.

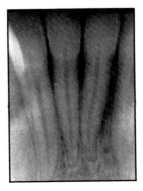 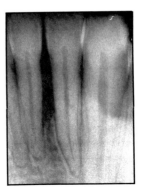

73, 74

The height and the course of the marginal bone crest can be observed from the radiographs. In periodontal health, the distance between the cementoenamel junction and the bone crest amounts to 1-1.5 mm. A layer of compact bone (lamina dura) may be observed lining the alveolar bone and following the root contours (Fig. 73, p. 76). The horizontal component of lamina dura interdentally may disappear in early periodontitis. However, the presence or absence of lamina dura is not a reliable sign of periodontitis due to variations in X-ray projection and the resulting images.

Periodontal bone height gradually reduces as periodontitis progresses (Fig. 74, p. 76; Fig. 76a-76d, p. 78). The bone loss should be analyzed for the various aspects of each tooth. The following questions should be asked: is the bone loss generalized or is it localized to a number of teeth? Is the pattern of bone loss horizontal or vertical? Are there intraosseous defects, furcation involvement and root concavities or furrows? Are there areas of calculus and overhanging restorations? Are the periodontal ligament spaces widened?

Lamina dura

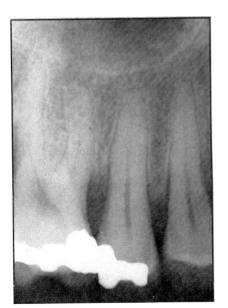 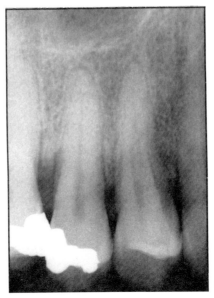

Fig. 75a, 75b. Radiographs from the same region, with somewhat different X-ray projection. The root concavity and the intraosseous defect (?) at the mesial aspect of the 1st premolar can be discerned from one of the radiographs (75b), but not from the other (75a). The marginal bone at the distal aspect of the 2nd premolar is also more clearly depicted in Fig. 75b.

75a, 75b

Combined clinical and radiographic examination

The evaluation of the radiographic images can be difficult. For example, intraosseous defects and furcation involvements may be masked by superimposition of dense bone or root structures (Fig. 64, p. 69; Fig. 65, p. 70). An intraosseous defect located at the buccal or at the lingual aspect of a tooth may be particularly difficult to detect. Inadequate angulation during X-ray projection may distort the appearance and the location of the marginal bone, complicating the analysis. A combination of careful clinical and radiographic examination is required for a successful evaluation.

Fig. 76a-76d. Bite-wing radiographs from the same patient, spanning a 5-year time interval (76a, 76b and 76c, 76d respectively). Calculus can be seen for several approximal surfaces at both time points. Additional loss of bone seems to have taken place at the mandibular left 1st molar, and at the mandibular right 1st and 2nd molars.

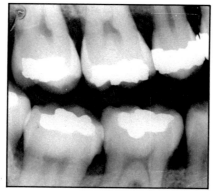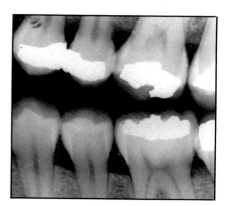

76a, 76b

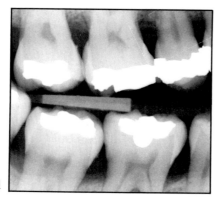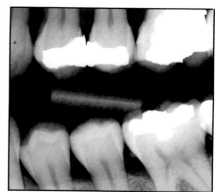

76c, 76d

Radiographic evaluation

Questions

1. What kinds of radiographic techniques may be used for the identification of periodontitis?

2. Why is X-ray projection important for periodontal diagnostic purposes?

3. Describe the radiographic appearance of healthy, marginal periodontal bone.

4. List the difficulties involved in reading radiographs for periodontal diagnostic purposes.

5. List the findings of interest one may encounter in radiographs of a periodontitis patient.

Explanation of terms

A

Acellular
not containing cells

Alveolar
pertaining to the alveolus

Alveolus
pl. alveoli, socket in the jaw
bone for anchorage of teeth

Amputation
removal of a limb (or root of a
tooth)

Anastomosis
connection between blood vessels

Anatomy
structure of the body

Anterior
situated in front

Antibody
molecule of the immune (defense) system that interacts
with an antigen

Antigen
noxious substance capable of
inducing an immune response

Antiseptic
substance that inhibits
microorganisms

Aperture
opening

Apex
tip (such as of a root)

Apical, apico-
towards or at the apex

Approximal
situated close together (such
as tooth surfaces facing a
neighboring tooth)

B

Bifurcation
site for division into two
branches (such as where the
trunk of a tooth separates into
two roots)

Bite-wing film
radiographic film hold by the
patient between the teeth, providing images of the crowns
and the upper and lower bone
crests

Bone marrow
soft tissue in cavities of the
bone

Bruxism
grinding and clenching of
teeth

Bucca
cheek

Buccal, bucco-
towards the cheek

C

Calcification
deposition of calcium salts

Calculus
abnormal deposit of mineral
salts (such as on the teeth)

Cancellous bone
bone with a lattice-like structure

Capillary
smallest type of blood vessel

Cavity
hollow space

Cellular
pertaining to a cell

Cementum
bone-like tissue covering the
roots of teeth

Cementocyte
cell in the cementum

Cementoenamel junction
border between the crown and
the root of teeth

Cervical
towards or at the cervix

Cervix
the neck or a constricted part
of an organ (such as a tooth)

Circumferential
pertaining to circumference

Col
a valley-like depression of the
interdental gengiva

Collagen
protein substance of the connective tissue fibers

Compact bone
dense, superficial bone layer

Connective tissue
tissue forming the supporting
and connecting structures of
the body

Corona
crown

Coronal
towards or at the crown

Corpuscle
small mass or body (such as a
red blood cell)

Crevice
longitudinal fissure

Crevicular
towards or at the crevice

Curet, curette
spoon-shaped instrument

Curettage
removal of material from a
cavity or a surface

Cuspid
canine tooth

Cyanosis
bluish discoloration of tissue
due to lack of oxygen

D

Debridement
removal of foreign material or
contaminated tissue from a
wound

Decalcification
dissolution and loss of calcium
salts

Degeneration
deterioration

Degradation
splitting or dissolution of a
substance

Dehiscence
split opening

Demineralization
see decalcification

Dens
tooth

Dental, dento-
pertaining to tooth

Dentin
the body of hard tissue of teeth
inside the enamel (crown) and
the cement (root)

Dentition
upper and lower teeth

Diastema
pl. diastemata, space between
two adjacent teeth

Disintegration
disruption, decomposing

Distal, disto-
position farther from the
median line of the jaw

Drainage
evacuation of fluids from a
wound or cavity

Dura
hard

E

Edema
excessive fluid in tissues

Elastic fibers
fibers present in some connective tissues (such as oral
mucosa)

Elongation
increasing or protruding in
length

Enamel
hard, glazed coat on the
crowns of teeth

Epithelium
pl. epithelia, tissue covering
all surfaces of the body

Erosion
an eating away

Eruption
appearing, breaking out

Erythema
redness

Exudate
fluid or cells escaped from
blood vessels

F
Facial, facio-
towards the face

Fenestration
window-like opening

Fiber
thread-like structure

Fibroblast
connective tissue cell producing collagen fibers

Fissure
cleft

Flap
partially removed piece of tissue

Fragility
lack of resistance to disruption

Frenulum
pl. frenula, fold of mucous
membranes

Fundus
bottom, base

Furcation
site for division into branches
(such as where the trunk of a
tooth separates into the roots)

G
Gingiva
"gum"

Gingivectomy
surgical removal of the gingiva

Gingivitis
inflammation of the gingiva

Ground substance
substance embedding cells and
fibers in the connective tissue

H
Hexagonal
having six sides

Histology
science of the minute tissue
structures

Hyper-
above, excessive

Hyperkeratinization
excessive presence of keratin

Hyperplasia
abnormal increase in the number of cells in the tissue

I
Immunology
science of the response of the
organism to antigenic chal-
lenge

Incisor
front tooth

Index
pl. indices, grading system

Infiltration
penetration or accumulation in
a tissue of cells or substances
not normal to it

Infra-
beneath

Infrabony
beneath the normal bone level

Inter-
between

Interdental
between the approximal surfaces of adjacent teeth

Interference
hampering of a procedure

Intra-
within

Intraosseous
within the bone

K
Keratin
protein substance of horny tissues

Keratinization
development of keratin

L
Lacuna
pl. lacunae, cavity

Lamella
pl. lamellae, thin leaf or plate
or layer, as of bone

Lamina
pl. laminae, thin, flat plate or layer

Lateral
position farther from the midline

Lesion
discontinuity of a tissue

Leukocyte
white blood cell

Ligament
band of fibrous tissue

Lingual, linguo-
towards the tongue

Lymphocyte
white blood cell, part of the lymphatic and immune systems

Lysis
dissolution, decomposition

M

Macrophage
large tissue cell capable of phagocytosis

Mandible
lower jaw

Margin
edge

Marginal
towards the margin

Marrow
see bone marrow

Mastication
chewing food

Matrix
pl. matrices, groundwork for a structure

Maxilla
upper jaw

Melanin
substance forming dark pigment

Melanocyte
cell producing melanin

Membrane
thin layer

Mesial, mesio-
towards the midline

Mineralization
see calcification

Molar
tooth positioned in the back of the mouth

Monocyte
white blood cell with one nucleus (kernel)

Morphology
science of the structure of organisms

Mucosa
see mucous membrane

Mucosal, muco-
pertaining to the mucous membrane

Mucous membrane
membrane lining cavities of the body

Mucus
product of glands (such as salivary)

Multi
many

O

Occlusion
tooth contacts, bite

Occlusal adjustment
correction of occlusion by selective grinding of the teeth

Orthodontics
correction of the position of teeth

Oral, orally
pertaining to the mouth

Orifice
entrance to a cavity

Os
bone

Osseous
pertaining to bone

Overlap
horizontal overlap of upper compared with lower teeth

P

Palatal
pertaining to the palate

Panoramic radiograph
radiographic method simultaneously providing images of both jaws and all teeth

Papilla
pl. papillae, nipple-shaped projection

Pathology
science of disease

Pellicle
thin film

Periapical film
radiographic image of teeth including structures around the root tip

Periodontitis
inflammation of the periodontium

Periodontium
the tissues that invest or help to invest and support the teeth

Permeability
permitting passage of substances

Phagocytosis
ingestion of particles or bacteria by cells

Physiology
science of the functions of living organisms

Plaque
patch or flat area

Plasma cell
cells capable of producing antibody

Plexus
network

Polymorphonuclear leukocyte
white blood cell with several nuclei (kernels)

Posterior
situated in back of

Premolar
teeth positioned in front of the molars

Prognosis
forecast

Progression
process of spreading or becoming more severe

Proliferation
multiplication

Proximal
nearest to

Pseudo
false

Pus
fluid with white blood cells caused by inflammation

R
Radiograph
image of calcified structures produced by X-rays

Radiopaque
visible in radiographs due to absorption of X-rays

Recession
act of receding

Resorption
loss of substance

Retention
keeping in place

Rete pegs
meshwork of pegs

Rupture
disruption of tissue

S
Septum
partition

Serum
clear portion of a body fluid (such as blood)

Serumal
pertaining to serum

Squamous
scaly, plate-like

Status
state, condition

Stippling
spotted appearance

Stratified
disposed in layers

Sub-
under

Sulcus
groove, furrow

Super-
above

Superimposition
placement upon or over

Supra-
above

Suppuration
discharge of pus

T
Tonus
tension, firmness

Topography
description of an anatomical
region

Toxic
poisonous

Trabecula
pl. trabeculae, supporting
strand

Translucent
transmitting light without providing distinct images

Trauma
wound, injury

Trifurcation
site for division into three
branches (such as where the
trunk of a tooth separates into
three roots)

U
Ulcer
local defect of tissue from
sloughing or shedding

Ulceration
ulcer, development of an ulcer

V
Vas
vessel, canal for fluids

Vascular
pertains to vessel

Vestibulum
chamber at an entrance to a
cavity